MANAGING YOUR
HEADACHES

Springer
New York
Berlin
Heidelberg
Barcelona
Hong Kong
London
Milan
Paris
Singapore
Tokyo

MANAGING YOUR
HEADACHES

~

Mark W. Green, M.D.
Leah M. Green, M.D.

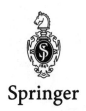

Springer

Mark W. Green, M.D.
Clinical Professor of Neurology
Columbia University College of Physicians and Surgeons
Headache Institute
St. Luke's–Roosevelt Hospital Center and Beth Israel Hospital Center
New York, NY 10019
USA

Leah M. Green, M.D.
Private Practice of Psychiatry
New York, NY 10019
USA

Library of Congress Cataloging-in-Publication Data
Green, Mark W.
Managing your headaches / Mark W. Green, Leah M. Green.
p. cm.
Includes bibliographical references and index.
ISBN 0-387-95238-1 (softcover : alk. paper)
1. Headache—Popular works. I. Green, Leah M. II. Title.
RC392.G74 2001
616.8′491—dc21   00-067909

Printed on acid free paper.

NOTE: The poem on page 2 is a Mesopotamian incantation dating from 4000–3000 B.C. It was found in a monograph by Arnold P. Friedman, M.D., entitled "Headache in History, Literature, and Legend," which was presented as a scientific exhibit at the 122nd Annual Convention of the American Medical Association, June 23–27, 1973, in New York City. Dr. Friedman was the first of five directors of the Montefiore Headache Unit. I was the second director, and he gave me this monograph in the late 1970s. —M.W.G.

Production managed by Steven Pisano; manufacturing supervised by Jacqui Ashri.
Composition by Matrix Publishing Services, Inc., York, PA.
Printed and bound by R.R. Donnelley and Sons, Harrisonburg, VA.
Printed in the United States of America.

9 8 7 6 5 4 3 2 1

ISBN 0-387-95238-1   SPIN 10793370

Springer-Verlag   New York Berlin Heidelberg
A member of BertelsmannSpringer Science+Business Media GmbH

To Stanley van den Noort, M.D., who told
me that if I went into neurosurgery rather
than neurology, he never would speak to me
again.

And to the late Elliott Weitzman, M.D.,
who had enough faith in me to allow me to
direct his wonderful headache unit.

M.W.G.

Contents

Introduction

During our past 22 years as a practicing neurologist specializing in headache (Dr. Mark Green) and a practicing psychiatrist (Dr. Leah Green), some important discoveries have improved the diagnosis and treatment of headache syndromes. These have proved enormously useful for management of headache. The value of this information increases when it is shared between physician and patient. Headache pain seems much less overwhelming when both parties understand its nature.

This book was written to give you the information you need to better manage your headaches. Understanding the causes and triggers of headache and the range of treatment options available will help you make good decisions about your care.

"Are you sure I don't have a brain tumor, Doctor?" is a common question for neurologists. Formerly, this concern was often the major reason for referral to a neurologist. Brain imaging was primitive then, and often painful and risky, whenever we decided to further investigate the cause of headaches. If no cause for the pain was discovered, the relieved patient then went back to the family doctor. The problem with this method was that neither physician appeared interested in dealing with the patient's pain, probably because the treatment options were discouragingly few.

With the medical technology available today, imaging has become easy and safe. Ruling out a brain tumor has become a simple matter. Patients no longer need a neurological examination; they need only place their heads in a scanning device.

There are two major difficulties with this solution: limited medical resources and limited benefit to the patient. Society simply can't afford the cost of supplying patients with a scan each time they experience a headache. The indication for brain imaging cannot be that the patient's insurance covers the test. More important, the overwhelming majority of headache sufferers don't need a scan and will receive no medical benefit whatsoever from undergoing one.

What is the alternative to this indiscriminate approach? It has continued to impress us through the years that taking a basic history and performing a physical examination remain the most important clinical techniques for every physician. The history of a patient's headaches and a careful neurological exam also help to reveal the diagnosis and direct the treatment. Little of importance is missed using these low-tech office procedures.

Once the patient and the doctor are able to rule out a brain tumor, the process of treating the headache syndrome begins. This must involve teaching the patient all the means in his power to treat himself.

The most difficult patients to treat are those who cannot provide accurate information about their headaches. This book will discuss the facts that should be recorded before consulting a headache specialist.

In the following chapters we will share our thought processes when evaluating patients and answering their questions. What should worry a headache sufferer and what should not? What is important to tell the doctor? What facts are known about headache and what remains to be discovered? What new treatment options are available? Can headaches be prevented?

Information is of the utmost importance in treatment. People can't manage their headaches without accurate information, and not all of it is simple to understand. They also need the support and understanding of their families, friends, and co-workers. Spouses and employers often misunderstand headaches. Those who suffer chronic (recurrent) headaches may feel that their lives are being controlled by their attacks. They are told that the problem is due to stress that they should be able to handle. This criticism causes loss of self-esteem at home and reduced productivity in the workplace. Caregivers also lose time at their jobs. Fear of severe headache drives sufferers to overmedicate themselves, particularly when they discover, as with some older drug treatments, that they do not work reliably. Leisure time is often adversely affected, as well as time with family and friends. The ability to limit the suffering and increase control over the attacks will improve the quality of life both for headache sufferers and those who live with them.

1

Headache for History Buffs

It seems particularly difficult for headache sufferers to accept the idea that "it's all in their heads." Most people find this hard to believe, especially when lying in bed in a dark room desperately trying not to vomit. Other theories of the cause of headache prevailed in the past, and it is interesting to speculate whether sufferers ever believed these explanations.

Primitive medicine originated from magical and religious beliefs. Early medical treatments applied not to mind or body alone but always to both. This approach gave healers the best outcomes. Ceremonies, prayers, chants, and sacred dances coupled with massage, sweat baths, purgatives, and incense inhalants relieved psychological and physical symptoms. Drugs received their healing power from the incantations that accompanied their administration. Add physical manipulation and the treatment had an even greater chance of success.

Headache has clearly existed at least as long as mankind. The first written descriptions of head pain date from Mesopotamian tablets of 4000 B.C. Demons were commonly thought to be the cause. An early description of the evil headache spirit, Ti'u, chasing a victim through the desert shows the power attributed to this illness.

Headache roameth over the desert, blowing like the wind,
Flashing like lightning, it is loosed above and below;
It cutteth off him who feareth not his god like a reed,
Like a stalk of henna it slitteth his thews.
It wasteth the flesh of him who hath no protecting goddess,
Flashing like a heavenly star, it cometh like the dew;
It standeth hostile against the wayfarer, scorching him like the day,
This man it hath struck and
Like one with heart disease he staggereth,
Like one bereft of reason he is broken,
Like that which has been cast into the fire he is shrivelled,

Like a wild ass . . . his eyes are full of cloud,
On himself he feedeth, bound in death;
Headache whose course like the dread windstorm none knoweth,
None knoweth its full time or its bond.

An exorcism was definitely in order for this unfortunate soul who had angered the gods. The priest-physician would use charms and amulets during the ceremony in combination with an ointment of human bone reduced to ashes mixed with cedar oil. Unpleasant substances were also applied. These treatments were to placate the spirits and persuade the headache to move elsewhere.

Other descriptions are more reminiscent of modern headache classifications. In this case it might have been a cluster variant: "a man's brain contains fire and myalgia afflicts the temples and smites the eyes, his eyes are afflicted with dimness, cloudiness, a disturbed appearance, with the veins bloodshot, shedding tears," or migraine: "when his brow pains a man and he vomits and is sick, his eyes being inflamed." Here the cause is thought to be the "hand of a ghost."

Egyptian gods such as Horus and Ra were known to suffer headaches. The goddess Isis treated Ra with a potion of coriander, wormwood, juniper, honey, and opium. A dancing girl in Pharaoh's court is mentioned in the Eber's papyrus as presenting with unilateral (one-sided) headaches accompanied by vomiting and malaise. This does sound like a description of migraine. Treatments employed by Egyptian physicians included trephining, which consisted of boring a hole in the skull "that the evil air may breathe out." Local remedies consisted of wet, cold mortar pressed to the scalp, or clay crocodiles bearing the names of the gods were bound firmly to the patient's head with linen strips. These may have compressed the superficial temporal arteries (those arteries that pound and ache during a migraine) and given relief. Modern-day preindustrial societies still trephine skulls to relieve chronic headache.

In 400 B.C. the Greek physician Hippocrates was the first to suggest that the cause of headache was other than the anger of the gods. He believed head pain occurred when the different elements of nature were out of harmony: blood, phlegm, black and yellow bile. This is called the humoral theory of illness. Pain resulted from vapors rising to the head from a bilious liver, and rational treatment consisted of bloodletting or applying herbs to the scalp to drain the excess liquids.

The Navaho people today employ ancient ceremonies to cure disease. As did Hippocrates, they believe that the sufferer needs to reintegrate into harmony with nature but with the help of family and friends. The cause of the illness may be a broken taboo or some offense to the gods. During the ceremony, the gods are persuaded to forgive the transgression. Purgatives, emetics, and sweat baths are physical treatments applied while the gods hear chants and view the sand paintings offered as appeasement for misdeeds. This method demonstrates how effective it may be to treat both mind and body.

We give credit to Hippocrates for realizing that there are different kinds of headaches, such as those associated with fever or infection, as opposed to a primary headache mentioned in the following description. "He seemed to see something shining before him like a light, usually in part of the right eye; at the end of a moment, a violent pain supervened in the right temple, then in all the head and neck . . . vomiting, when it became possible, was able to divert the pain and render it more moderate." This patient appears to have migraine symptoms including a visual aura prior to the headache.

Four hundred years later, Aretaeus of Cappadocia (A.D. 30–90) classified three distinct types of headache, including one called "heterocrania," the set of symptoms now called migraine. This type of headache lasted from 6 to 24 hours and consisted of one-sided throbbing head pain, gastric upset, and sensitivity to light, sound, and smells. Aretaeus proposed treatment based on the theory that counterirritants would dispel the headache. Substances such as pitch were smoothed on a shaved head to raise blisters and rid the sufferer of internal head pain.

In Roman times the physician Galen (A.D. 131–201) used the Greek word "hemicrania" (meaning half the head) to describe these headaches. This translated to the Latin "hemicranium," eventually becoming "emigranea" and then "mygraine" and "megrim" in English. These terms refer to the "sick headaches" of migraine. Interested in anatomy and influenced by the writings of Hippocrates, Galen thought the cause was bilious vapors to the brain carried by blood vessels from the body. To treat these attacks, he prescribed bloodletting and application of local cold packs. He also believed counterirritants to be useful and advocated placing a live electric fish, called a torpedo, on the forehead. As did the Egyptian gods, Galen also treated with narcotics such as opium and mandragora.

The importance of trigger factors in precipitating migraine was documented by the Roman, Celsus (25 B.C. to A.D. 50) who mentioned "wine, cold, heat of fire, or the sun" could bring on a headache. He wrote that migraine was not fatal and had an episodic and chronic nature throughout one's life span.

Headache is mentioned in the Talmud, a collection of rabbinical discussions of biblical law compiled during the second through sixth centuries, as caused by blowing away the foam of drinks like beer or mead. Again, alcohol is noted as a trigger. There was also a belief that headache comes from committing sins and may be cured by penitence and the performance of good works. Rubbing the head with wine, vinegar, or oil was also recommended. Moses Maimonides, physician and spiritual leader of the Egyptian Jewish community of the twelfth century, believed, as did Galen, that headaches were due to disequilibrium of body humors, and championed preventive medicine such as healthy diet and exercise to treat illness. Specific remedies included binding the temples, bloodletting from the pulsing arteries behind the ears, and vomiting twice a month to purge the system.

During the Middle Ages, there was little change from the Greco-Roman school of thought about the causes and treatment of headache. Several physicians did record the details of their personal migraine attacks. One of these was Felix Wuertz of Switzerland, who also described cutting off blood flow in the superficial temporal artery, the blood vessel that throbs in your temple, as a beneficial treatment.

The first to mention headache as a symptom of occupational illness was Bernardo Ramazzini in his treatise "De morbis artificum diatriba," published in 1700 at the University of Modena. Twelve professions are listed, including pharmacists; oil-miller, tanners, and other grimy craftsmen; tobacco workers; wet nurses; brewers of alcoholic beverages; tailors; wool carders; runners; scribes and stenographers; confectioners sugar coating seeds over burning coals; carpenters; sailors and galley slaves; and hunters. Ramazzini believed the cause of headache for the majority of these professions was the inhalation of noxious vapors and, in the case of coal, a toxic carbon oxide gas. For desk workers and seamstresses, he attributed their suffering to long hours of intense attention under wretched environmental conditions, resembling a modern tension headache. Sailors and hunters appeared to react to changes in temperature and sun exposure. The headache of wet-nurses arose from fatigue associated with sleep disturbance. Some professions worsen headaches in those who already have the problem, such as singers and musicians who must contract abdominal and pectoral muscles, affecting the flow of blood to the head. Suggested cures include removal of noxious odors and better workplace hygiene. For pharmacists, he wrote "Those in whom the power of scent of dogs resides should run away from such smells as far as possible, and again and again go out of the shop to breath fresh air, or very often hold more welcome scents to their noses, by which they may regularly obtain relief, and blunt the offending smells." Consideration of headache triggers in the workplace is important to modern management of this illness.

The next advance occurred in seventeenth-century England with the vascular theory of Dr. Thomas Willis. He stated that the pain of megrim originated from swollen blood vessels expanding in the head, explaining the throbbing quality of the pain. He further suggested that there is also a disturbance originating in the brain during the headache. No techniques were available at that time to prove his theory. It was not until the 20th century that Dr. Harold Wolff demonstrated this finding during actual migraine attacks. Willis used ointment of quicksilver, mercurial powder, and spaw-waters to treat headache, but admitted that "For the obtaining a Cur, or rather for a tryal very many Remedies were administered, thorow the whole progress of the Disease, by the most skilful Physicians . . . without any success or ease. . . ."

In the late 1700s, Erasmus Darwin, physician and grandfather of naturalist Charles Darwin, also proposed that migraine headaches were due to dilating (enlarging) blood vessels in the brain and tried a logical cure. Patients were spun in a large centrifuge to force blood from the head to the feet and relieve the swelling. This probably did result in patient well-being when the spinning finally stopped.

During the next two centuries, physicians described many different factors influencing the development of headaches. These included diet, underlying psychological difficulties, ovarian influences, and gastrointestinal disturbances. Dr. Edward Liveing wrote "On Megrim, Sick-Headache, and Some Allied Disorder," in 1873, describing general faulty habits of life as causing the illness. He recommended improvement in diet, restoring health through rest and good hygiene, as well as sedatives like belladonna or tonics like iron and quinine.

Toward the end of the 1800s, exploration of the causes of common headaches such as tension-type became the focus of physicians. Victorian neurologists thought the cause was thinking too heavily, hysteria, or hypochondria. Treatments ran the gamut from bed rest to vigorous exercise. Medicines included laudanum and hemp. Sigmund Freud, physician and founder of modern psychoanalysis, wrote that the logical center for migraine "is a trigeminal nucleus whose fibers supply the dura matter" and "may include spastic innervation of muscles of blood vessels in the reflex sphere of the dural region." This anticipated the current theory of Moskowitz that abnormally dilated meningeal vessels (blood vessels on the outside of the brain) produce nerve signals that stimulate trigeminovascular nerves to produce migraine.

The twentieth-century physician William Osler first introduced the idea that the muscles of the head were abnormally tense during this headache. Wolff studied this and showed that involuntary contraction of scalp and neck muscles does cause headache. He called this "muscle-contraction" headache. More recent studies show no consistent correlation between this headache and muscle contraction. A unifying theory of headache now accepted by many physicians supports the idea that migraines and tension headaches are part of a continuum and actually may shift from one to another.

Understanding the causes of headache has brought a new direction in effective treatment. Documentation of changes during the migraine attack has led to current therapies with ergots to shrink blood vessels. More recent evidence of local arterial wall inflammation with dropping serotonin levels has led to the development of drugs like dihydroergotamine and sumatriptan.

Misery loves company, and it might make us feel better to know that many famous persons also suffered from headache. Among them are former U.S. presidents Ulysses S. Grant and

Thomas Jefferson; writers Guy de Maupassant, Edgar Allan Poe, Leo Tolstoi, Virginia Woolf, and Lewis Carroll; scientists Carl Linnaeus, Charles Darwin, and Sigmund Freud; philosophers Immanuel Kant and Karl Marx; Roman Emperor Julius Caesar, Mary Todd Lincoln and Madame de Pompadour.

Throughout the past, and certainly into the future, headache research continues to advance, giving us greater knowledge that will help us to develop rational, safer, and more effective treatments. It is clearly important not to lose sight of the powerful effect of addressing these remedies to both the mind and the body.

2

Maybe I Have a Sinus Headache

In Chapter 1, we described historical beliefs and treatments for headache. Now we will explore modern beliefs that may be no more accurate.

Common Beliefs About Headache Causes

This first belief is that chronic sinus disease is a common cause of headache. Millions of dollars each year in the United States are spent on sinus medications. Lots of people are convinced that this is what troubles them. The advertisements for sinus pills list symptoms that anyone with any kind of headache can relate to; most headache sufferers can probably be convinced to try the pills.

Many receive sinus x-rays as part of their headache evaluation. Frequently, the reports return showing the "chronic changes" of sinusitis, often on one side. The problem is that, just as often, the changes are on the side opposite the headache. Periodically we see people getting surgical procedures to treat these changes on the x-ray. This rarely helps.

There are two kinds of sinusitis: **acute sinusitis** and **chronic sinusitis**. The acute kind is just that: an acute illness, often with fever and a lot of tenderness over the sinuses and frequently an infected drainage coming from the nose. The pain you get is generally felt as a deep ache located over the affected sinus. Leaning forward commonly increases the pain, but that is true of migraine and other types of headaches as well. Your sinuses feel blocked, but sinus congestion may occur with migraine and particularly with cluster headaches. In those cases, the sensation of fullness in the sinus is the headache, not its cause.

The important point to realize is that no one walks around for months or years with acute sinusitis before it comes to medical attention because it is an acute disorder that makes people very ill. If you do have acute sinusitis, you should not just take sinus medicines; at the minimum, you need antibiotics and medical attention.

Chronic sinusitis is different. It seems that this is a rare cause of headaches, even though chronic sinusitis is common. It certainly never causes you to be fine for days and weeks, then suddenly become very ill for hours, then well again.

The same is true for eyeglasses. Eyestrain rarely causes severe headache. When it does, it is clearly related to reading or getting new glasses. Needing corrective lenses or a stronger prescription will not cause you to be very sick every once in a while, then fine for the rest of the time. If reading brings on your headaches, check that out with your eye doctor.

Everyone is allergic to something, and it is another misconception that allergies are an important cause of headaches. If you have migraine, you might expect to see an increase in your migraines when you are in an allergic period, just as you might with any stress. But focusing the treatment of your headache problem on allergies is not likely to be fruitful. In Chapter 6 we will talk about foods that can trigger migraines. These foods don't produce migraines on the basis of allergy, however, so allergy shots won't protect you against migraines.

A 23-year-old woman complains of pain in her left temple and in front of her left ear. She notes that if she chews, the pain becomes worse, and she has been eating soft foods. She has felt very stressed, and her sleep is disturbed. The pain is described as an ache, and she doesn't otherwise feel sick with this headache.

Many people have, or believe they have, **temporomandibular joint (TMJ) dysfunction** as the cause of their headaches. This is a syndrome that causes discomfort when you chew. There is a large muscle in the temples, the temporalis muscle, which can be in spasm. When you open your mouth, a click may be noted in or around the ear. Other muscles in and around the mouth may also be involved. TMJ dysfunction doesn't always mean that there is a problem with the joint. Often the joint dislocates as part of a tension-type headache where the muscles are putting a lot of pressure on the joint. Very often, people with this kind of headache grind their teeth or clench their jaws often while they sleep.

Most of us have had this problem from time to time. Studies show that 75% of the population will have a TMJ disorder at some time or another. Often it will occur if you yawn widely or open your mouth and bite into a candy apple or a tough piece of meat. Usually that will go away in a few minutes or at least in a day or so. But there are a few poor souls who develop this as a chronic problem.

Some anti-inflammatory medicines and a mild muscle relaxant may suffice as treatment for those with an acute TMJ disorder. If it becomes chronic, you need to see your dentist to determine whether there is a problem in the joint or whether there is something wrong with your bite. Occasionally your dentist may want you to wear an appliance to equilibrate your bite or at least keep you from grinding your teeth down. Periodically, surgical management is recommended. This should be reserved only for unusual situations where the diagnosis of TMJ dysfunction is absolutely certain and all other treatment approaches have been exhausted.

The Primary Headache Syndromes

Let's get to the most likely causes of your headache. There is no such thing as a "regular headache." Studies have shown that 90% of all chronic, recurring headaches are either migraine or tension-type headaches. So we had better understand what these are. When we, as physicians, look at chronic and recurring headaches, there are literally hundreds of causes. That means that only 10% of people with chronic recurring headaches have any of the other hundreds of causes. Most of those other causes are **secondary headaches**, as opposed to migraine, tension-type headache, and cluster, which are the **primary headache syndromes**.

It frequently comes as quite a surprise to people when they are told they have migraine. Studies have shown that there are 21.1 million migraine sufferers in the United States. Only 11.2 million are diagnosed, leaving slightly less than half of migraineurs unidentified. Men are less likely to be diagnosed than women. This arises from the misconception that men don't get migraine. This results in failure to find an effective treatment.

Studies show that patients try nearly five treatment options before finding one that works, and spend, on average, $3^{1}/_{2}$ years to find that successful treatment.

Migraine headaches usually begin in childhood, typically worsening until around age 40 before they begin to improve. This pattern is very different from most other afflictions, which increase in likelihood in the elderly. Migraine is most prevalent during the years that people are ordinarily most productive in their careers and in raising their families. That is another reason why the disability of migraine is so costly. While you are reading these words, over 1 million Americans will be suffering from migraine. Of these, 61% of the attacks will last 3 to 12 hours, and 12% will last longer than a day. In addition to the personal suffering of 30 million headache patients and their families, migraines also result in over 6 billion lost working days and 74 million days of restricted activity yearly. Over 3 million days per month are spent bedridden. If you have migraine, you are likely to have a lot of attacks, with the average person experiencing three and a half attacks monthly. All of this translates to $17 billion in lost income and productivity. If you include the cost of caring for these attacks and their related health problems, the economic burden for society becomes closer to $50 billion annually.

It is expensive to have migraine. Your missed work and impaired functioning during an attack mean that you are a less desirable employee (statistically; we're not pointing fingers). When it comes to promotions and raises, people with migraine fare poorly. Migraine sufferers have lower incomes than those without this problem.

Statistics on lost working days don't tell us how migraine affects the quality of life for sufferers. Experts now have tools to measure these impact data and have applied it to this population. The results are astounding. Quality of life can be formally measured in various medical conditions. The quality of life for those with migraine is poor even when compared to other chronic disorders. Scores were worse for migraine than for depression, back problems, recent heart attack, and congestive heart failure. Only active AIDS scored worse.

What symptoms do you get when you develop a migraine? Many migraines begin with a **prodrome**, which often occurs well before the attack begins, even the day before. If you can identify a prodrome in yourself, you may be able to get a big jump on treatment of your attack.

Prodromes are often very subtle. Until they are pointed out, you probably won't realize you have one. Common prodromes include mental changes. Depression is particularly common, but, interestingly, **euphoria** (a positive, happy mood) is even more common. Many people feel particularly well before their migraine begins. Irritability and restlessness can certainly occur and yawning is an interesting behavior that often heralds the onset of a migraine. We find that spouses are often better than patients in appreciating that yawning is going to lead to a headache. Other prodromal symptoms can include neck stiffness, which may be the earliest sign of the headache to follow. Cold hands and feet are common migraine prodromes. We've known that migrainous people tend to have cold hands and feet even between attacks. The extremities become increasingly cold during the attack. This observation is what led to the development of biofeedback, teaching people to change skin temperature of their hands as a migraine treatment. You may already be familiar with the idea of food cravings and food aversions commonly associated with pregnancy. Migraine sufferers don't want pickles and ice cream, but they may want other foods. These cravings are neurobiologically mediated and commonly occur with migraines as well.

One of the food cravings we've become most interested in is the craving for chocolate. Many people believe that chocolate triggers migraines. However, this is controversial since several studies have thrown a monkey wrench into this thought. They failed to prove that when migraineurs were given chocolate versus placebo you could predict who would get migraines. There is evidence that a chocolate craving may simply be a migraine prodrome. If you understand this, you can realize that a craving for chocolate is going to herald the onset of a migraine. When you act upon it and eat chocolate, you blame the chocolate for triggering a migraine. Instead, it may simply be part of the attack. To be fair, other studies have suggested chocolate to be an actual trigger for some attacks.

Migraine is the most important headache type. In the past, we used to divide migraine into two groups, **classic** and **common migraine**. In 1988, experts got together to reclassify headaches. They published the classification we now use, the International Headache Society or IHS classification.

A 27-year-old woman came to my office complaining about a one-sided pounding headache from which she awakened each Saturday morning. It usually involved the right side of her head, but occasionally was left sided or involved both sides. The right-sided ones were always the worst ones, and within an hour she would get a great deal of nausea. If she had wine with dinner, the headaches seemed worse, but they would occur frequently without drinking. She told me she thought that she must be allergic to alcohol. She was bothered by lights and sounds, but found that the pain was worse if she didn't get out of bed and shower. The

*headache usually improved by the evening, but never went away
completely until she slept the next night.*

When we were in medical school we were told that there
are two kinds of migraine: classic migraine and common migraine. The current terminology no longer uses those terms.
We now refer to **migraine with aura** and **migraine without
aura**. Migraine without aura comprises about 85% of migraine
attacks. The pain of migraine is usually on one side, but can
be two sided. Both-sided headaches with migraines are particularly likely to occur in children. The pain of migraine tends
to be pounding in quality. If it isn't pounding when you are
standing, just lean forward and you will appreciate the pul-
satile quality of the pain. Finally, it tends to worsen with movement and if you exert yourself it will further increase the pain.
We are uncomfortable about making the diagnosis of migraine
with certainty when there have only been one or two attacks.
But when the attacks become recurrent, the chance of the
headache being migrainous is more likely. The term migraine
comes from "megrim," and migraines are indeed "sick"
headaches. By sick we mean that migraines are often associated with nausea, vomiting, light sensitivity, and sound sensitivity. When you get a migraine, you don't want to smell dinner cooking and you want to be in a quiet, dark place.

*A 17-year-old boy complained that when he was playing base-
ball in the sun, he suddenly developed a shimmering light on the
right side of his vision. Over the next 20 minutes, as the flashing light got larger, he noted that he couldn't see the right side
of his coach's face. He was relieved that it went away in a half
hour, until he developed a pounding headache behind his left eye
and began to vomit.*

Migraine with aura causes the same headache and associated symptoms that we just described, now preceded by some type of neurological event. We used to speak only about **visual auras** when we used the term classic migraine, but under the present terminology all auras are lumped together as migraine with aura. Numbness on one side of the body, inability to find words or speak (**aphasia**), or an actual paralysis on one side of the body, may all be considered migraine with aura. But the most common auras are still visual illusions of varying types. The visual auras generally last about 20 minutes, although some last up to an hour. Their onset is generally gradual (over a few minutes), and they often begin with a small blind spot or disturbance of vision, which enlarges over time. Patients feel that this is a problem in their eye, but that is rarely the case. The problem is, in fact, located in parts of the brain that subserve vision; therefore, both eyes are generally involved equally. When you look out into space you will likely see the disturbance in one side of the room, but this persists even if you cover one eye or the other. This is because each eye duplicates each visual field. Migraine auras often have two components. The first is something we refer to as a **positive neurological phenomenon**; this is often bright and flashing. The second component is called a **negative neurological phenomenon**, which is a blind spot. An example is **fortification spectra**, common visual auras of a C-shaped, zigzag outline. The lead edge of this outline is often shimmering. As it enlarges over the hour, it often leaves a blind spot behind it. Visual aura can be seen as bright flashing lights, or one entire visual field on the left or right side can be missing or impaired. Vision can break down into cubes or small pieces of vision. Sometimes the visual disturbances are particularly frightening, and images can be moving. On other occasions objects can become very large, very small, or very distorted. This is what we believe Lewis Carroll may have experienced, and we often refer to this as the Alice in Wonderland syndrome.

Sometimes the aura occurs and no headache follows. We call these **acephalic migraines**. These are particularly likely to occur in the elderly. If you have a long history of migraine with auras, then begin to experience only the auras, the attacks are still migraines although treatment is not usually necessary.

The auras do go away, and usually a headache follows. The headache fulfills the criteria just described: a pounding, one-sided or two-sided headache accompanied by nausea, vomiting, light sensitivity, and sound sensitivity. You don't need all of these symptoms to call it a migraine. Even if you have all of these symptoms with your attacks and have regular headaches in between, the regular headaches are likely to be mild migraines.

Other auras are even more frightening, but are, fortunately, relatively rare. A syndrome called **ophthalmoplegic migraine** involves changes in the pupils and movements of the eye. Another variant of migraine with aura is called **basilar migraine**. Here, people may have double vision, difficulty in swallowing or speaking, dizziness, weakness or numbness on one or two sides of the body, as well as confusion or lethargy. They may feel that they are walking like a drunk; they may become sleepy or, on rare occasions, even become comatose.

An 8-year-old boy came home from school once or twice a month complaining of stomachache. He would open his windows, turn off the lights, and sleep for an hour. Periodically, he would vomit. After an hour of sleep, he awakened hungry and ready for dinner.

It is a myth that children don't get headaches. Unfortunately, children do have headaches, particularly migraine. Migraine is a familial disease. That means that if you have migraine, there is a fair chance that your kids are going to have migraine. We don't like to think that we gave something bad to our children. Of course, we give them some of our good traits as well. Another reason to understand this material is to help our children gain a better understanding of this problem.

We often don't recognize migraines when they first occur because migraines in childhood don't have to include head pain. Remember that migraine is a brain disorder and lots of brain symptoms can be part of the syndrome. One hint that migraine is present in childhood is the symptom of carsickness. A high percentage of migrainous kids are carsick. When they grow up we eventually recognize that they have migraine. Many children will come home from school from time to time looking pale, nauseated, and very fatigued. They fall asleep and then awaken an hour later feeling fine. That event could be a migraine, even if there was no headache. Spells of abdominal (stomach) pains can be migrainous, and an ill-looking child returning home from school with a stomachache can have migraine.

A baby with repetitive spells of vomiting with no other cause found could have migraine. Unfortunately, there is no way of proving it at the time, but your pediatrician can suspect it. As the child grows up, it often becomes quite clear that the doctor was right as more typical migraine attacks are identified.

The other common type of primary headache syndrome is called a **tension-type headache**. This clumsy term has an interesting history. When we were in school, these were called *tension headaches*; however, doctors argued over what that meant. Some believed that the muscles were tense, while others who used this term believed the person was tense, so clearly the term *tension* was ambiguous. The experts then coined the term *muscle contraction headache*, which was a fine term explaining that what was tense were the muscles of the scalp and head. The problem is that many times tension headaches are not associated with any more tension than a nonheadache period. Furthermore, people with migraine seem to have as much tension in their muscles as do tension headache sufferers. But we all can agree that the syndrome exists.

> *A 58-year-old woman came in with headaches that she experienced at least four times each week. She described her pain as an ache throughout her head and shoulders. The attacks lasted all day. She didn't feel sick with these attacks, and she was able to function, but she described these as "annoying."*

Many people—over 50% of the population—experience **episodic tension-type headaches**. These are usually not a major problem and are often associated with a specific stress or some prolonged posture with the neck. A long car drive or a long time looking at a computer screen, or even the use of a new pillow, can trigger these headaches. The pain is on both sides of the head, often described as a "bandlike headache," or people feel as if they have a tight cap around their head. You don't get very sick with these, and you are generally not sleepy as part of the attack. They usually last a few hours and tend to be easily relieved, often with over-the-counter medications or just rest.

Chronic tension-type headaches are a much bigger problem, although fortunately, they are much rarer. In this syndrome, patients go from months to years without relief but have the same quality of pain just described. Many people who have these are depressed, but it doesn't mean that they are depressed simply because they have the headaches.

A 51-year-old woman states that she has had an ache through-
out her head for many years, and it rarely goes away. She can
"live with that," but every few weeks she has a headache that
seems the same as the others, then develops a throbbing quality
and settles behind her left eye. She becomes very tired and nau-
seated with those headaches, which take up to 2 days to resolve.

In 1988, the concept was proposed that tension-type
headaches and migraine represent in many ways the opposite
ends of the spectrum of a continuum of chronic recurring
headaches, and so reflect the same underlying process. In other
words, all of these headaches are related. Other headache experts
feel strongly that the terms *migraine* and *tension* need to be sep-
arated and are very different phenomena, with different causes.

Many people say that their migraines start out like tension
headaches and end up like migraines. Others say that their migraines wind up like tension headaches. It seems that a large
number of people have both, and there must be a close relationship between these two types of headaches. So, if you have
migraine and tension headaches, you may not actually have
two distinct types of headache. However, this does not mean
that they feel the same or even that they should be treated the
same way.

We have learned that people with migraine who experience different kinds of headaches often respond to one migraine medication for all their headaches. A recent study done
with Imitrex (sumatriptan) showed that these people re-
sponded well when they had typical migraines, typical tension
headaches, and those with features of each. It seems, therefore,
that in this setting we do best by choosing an agent based on
the severity of pain, rather than trying to distinguish the type
of headache. It is important to recognize that if you have re-

current disabling headaches, you are most likely suffering from migraine.

A 48-year-old man came into the office desperate for treatment of agonizing headaches that he had been experiencing over the past 2 weeks. Whenever he fell asleep, he was awakened by a severe pain behind his right eye. Attacks lasted 2 hours, and he had been getting one or two attacks each day. He noted that a clear liquid runs from his right nostril when he gets an attack and that his right eye tears as well. He was checked for sinusitis, but no significant abnormalities were found. Codeine didn't help relieve the pain.

This man has cluster headaches. Cluster headaches are a distinctive form of headache that shouldn't be confused with other kinds of headaches. These are really awful, but fortunately rare. They occur in fewer than one in a thousand people. The ratio of men to women with cluster headaches is 6 to 1. This is in contrast to migraine, which is three times more common in women.

Usually they occur in clusters, within a period that generally lasts 2 weeks to 2 months. Between these clusters, people are usually well. But as soon as a cluster period begins, it is clear that rough times are ahead. The usual cluster patient will have one or more headaches each day, day after day, lasting $1/2$ to 2 hours. These headaches are very painful, much more so than migraines. The pain usually begins in one temple or behind the eye, or the cheek or upper teeth. The pain builds up much more quickly than it does with migraine, usually over minutes. The eye on the side of the pain gets red and runs, and a clear liquid runs from the nose. This clear liquid often convinces the sufferers that the problem is in their sinuses, and the severe eye pain may drive them to see their eye doctor. Even the behavior of someone with cluster headaches is different from someone with migraine. Migraineurs want to go to bed and remain motionless. They want to squeeze their temples into their pillow and hold still. Cluster headache sufferers can't hold still. They rock, pace, and cry. Alcohol can trigger a migraine, but it is amazing how sensitive cluster headache sufferers are to drinking alcohol. A half glass of wine or a few sips of beer are likely to induce an agonizing attack during a cluster period. Even the minute amount of alcohol found in "nonalcoholic" beers can be enough. Sleep can trigger a migraine, but with cluster this is very common. You may be awakened from sleep, often at the same time every night. This feature led to an old term for cluster headaches, **alarm clock headaches**.

Even though alcohol triggers cluster headaches, it is astounding that over 50% of people with cluster headaches abuse alcohol, which is much more than the general population. Cluster headache sufferers usually smoke cigarettes as well. This is a big problem. Smoking may be a major mechanism for developing the problem in the first place through the effect of smoke on a ganglion of nerves in the back of the throat. Also, cigarette smoking puts these people at high risk of developing heart disease. Most of the effective medications for cluster cannot be used if you have heart disease that involves the arteries of the heart (coronary artery disease). Therefore smoking really limits our options for treating these terrible headaches.

Another interesting relationship with cluster is the increased risk of developing a stomach ulcer. If you have cluster headaches, particularly if you have cheek and tooth pains with the attacks, you are at high risk of developing this problem as well. Unfortunately, the medications used to treat the ulcer don't help the headaches.

3

Maybe It's All Due to Stress

Everyone has heard the explanation that headaches are caused by stress. Stress can certainly play a role in making any kind of headache worse, from a migraine to a brain tumor.

Headache and Stress

We don't think there really is something called a "stress headache." This is a catchall term, not in the vocabulary of a headache expert. It is tossed around as freely as the term "sinus headache." There is also nothing called a "regular headache." Each type of head pain has it own physiological basis.

Let's define stress. Individuals experience stress in different ways, according to their psychological makeup. What is stressful for one may not be stressful for another. Stress occurs when a person confronts a demand that he feels he cannot meet. The result is internal conflict, and stress continues until that conflict is resolved. The nature of those demands may vary widely among individuals. Situations that require a great deal of flexibility may exceed an individual's capacity to respond. In this way, they generate stress. One person may find vacations relaxing, while another feels unfamiliar activities are threatening. Others do best at work. Studies involving the role of stress in producing headache are difficult to interpret because the conditions used to precipitate stress may not have the same meaning for all individuals.

Reaction to stress that cannot be handled adequately may lead to events that occur in neuroreceptor pathways and trigger the headache process. The expectation of headache is then set and may actually increase its probability of occurring. These reactions will also influence the way we perceive pain. Perception is all that matters with pain. Nothing is intrinsically painful. It is how our brain perceives an event that translates into pain. Anxiety also increases when stress is not mastered, and this could lead to the worsening of anxiety syndromes that can be associated with headache.

Stress should be viewed as a headache trigger, but not the cause. The underlying individual genetic predisposition must exist for a situation in your life to activate these chemical pathways and ultimately to result in a headache. As with other triggers, proper management may lessen frequency and intensity of pain. Problem solving, seeking emotional supports, mastering new coping skills, and efforts to even the stress level over the day are all helpful in decreasing number and severity of attacks.

Stress is one of many headache triggers. Stress can also provoke other chronic pain responses such as increased heart rate, abdominal pain, muscle aches, and syndromes such as asthma attacks and ulcer pain. Those who experience migraine must have the underlying genetic makeup to experience headache as a result.

Better management of stress, as with management of other triggers, may reduce the number and severity of headaches. Diagnosis and treatment of accompanying psychiatric conditions such as depression and anxiety disorders also contribute to better headache control.

Dr. Sigmund Freud, founder of psychoanalysis and himself a migraine sufferer, wrote about his theories of chronic pain and migraine. The worst period of his attacks coincided with the stress he experienced while exploring internal conflicts during his own self-analysis. As he was able to resolve his conflicts, his headaches lessened. This applies to the treatment of migraine in modern times, and resolving conflicts still has a place in improving headache syndromes. His emphasis on understanding the individual meaning of pain through exploring each sufferer's psychological, social, and family history has great importance in the current treatment of headache. His observation that susceptibility to trigger factors depends on the level of stimulation already present in the individual helps to explain why the presence of a trigger does not always produce a headache.

Which are more stressful: hassles of daily living or major life events? Is peak stress more likely to cause headache or is a continuous stress level? How long after a stressful event does a headache occur?

Findings indicate that the headache comes about an hour or so after a stress peak while stress during the attack may increase the intensity of the pain. Continuous stress levels are handled better than changing levels. They require fewer changes in coping skills and less need for problem solving. Major life events, whether positive or negative, increase stress and can trigger a migraine. During an ongoing stress, patients may find they are protected from getting a headache. As soon as the stress is relieved, the headache arrives. College students who worry that they will get headaches during their exams usually feel well until the stress is over. This is the "letdown headache." Stress increases the perception of head pain, and efforts to keep a regular daily routine should help reduce both stress and headache.

Prospective scientific studies (those choosing subjects and following them forward in time) dealing with the relationship of stress and headache can't adequately reproduce the character of everyday stress in the experiment. For example, the task of multiplying numbers has been used as a stressor. Do headache sufferers report more daily hassles because they really occur, or is that simply how they view life? Retrospective studies (those that gather information about past headaches) generate answers affected by memory and influenced by personal prejudices about the causes of headache. It certainly does appear that stress is only one of many factors involved in the production of head pain and its variability. How might stress influence the development of headache? Responses to the stressful situation may cause harmful behaviors that predispose to head pain or help to maintain it.

Chronic Headache and Psychological Problems

For decades, it has been written that there is a "migraine personality." Classic descriptions of the migraine patient personality include anxiety, depression, hypochondria (excessive preoccupation with illness), rigidity, hostility, and resentment. These people were felt to be perfectionists. An overall view may be seen in the concept of neuroticism, a general emotional over-activity that may lead to psychological disorders under stress. This also predisposes an individual to overuse medications. Do anger and hostility increase headache or does living with chronic daily pain produce the anger and hostility? The idea of a specific migraine personality is probably flawed. It results from studies drawn on clinic-based patients who are a self-selected population of people more inclined to seek treatment. This can be caused by pre-existing traits or unusually severe headaches. Comorbidity (occurring together) of head pain and psychiatric disease is associated with seeking care for headache disorders and contributes to an overestimation of psychological syndromes found in clinic populations. Most likely is that migraine and certain types of psychiatric disorders share specific genetic and environmental risk factors. Complicated stuff!

Prospective studies have shown that subjects with migraine have more mood and anxiety disorders compared to those without migraine. Tension-type headache sufferers aren't any different from controls in rates of psychopathology or personality factors. Occurrence of anxiety disorders precedes migraine onset in 80% of patients with both conditions, while depression follows migraine in 75% of cases.

Recent epidemiological studies, based on community populations, suggest that there is an association between migraine and major depression as well as manic-depressive, anxiety, and panic disorders. This influence between migraine and depression is found to be bidirectional. That means that the presence of one disorder increases the risk of having the other. The best explanation is again the existence of another factor underlying these disorders and causing both. It's not that migraine causes you to be depressed or being depressed causes you to have migraines. A more likely explanation is that regulation of the serotonergic neurotransmitter system is impaired in both of these disorders. Migraine, chronic pain syndromes, major depressive syndromes, and anxiety and panic disorders all may respond to some antidepressant medications. These drugs work by increasing transmission at neurological junctions and may work on a common cause for both the headache and psychological disorders.

Migraine attacks challenge the ability to cope for many who are already emotionally overactive and may predispose them to depression and anxiety disorders. For women, the headaches increase as estrogen and progesterone fall, so they are worse during the premenstrual phase and better during ovulation. Correlating with this, the ability to cope is best at ovulation and worst in the premenstrual period.

Chronic pain sufferers are a varied group. Some are unaware of psychological problems, while others seek help. There are a wide variety of coping styles, but those that drive one to seek social support are more successful than those that end in social isolation. It is important to be aware that adolescents with chronic daily headache are at risk for depression and are often found to have a precipitating event such as loss of a family member, terminal illness in the family, separation of parents, or change of residence. In these cases psychological treatment with appropriate medication is necessary.

Frequent headaches tend to isolate people socially and affect their performance in their work environment. Loss of self-esteem and loss of self-control worsen the condition. Improvement in headache management can change this by itself, but if psychological problems persist, treatment can improve mental attitude and quality of life.

4

Are You Sure I Don't Have a Brain Tumor?

Almost every patient we see with headaches, whether they mention it or not, worries that we might be failing to diagnose their brain tumor. In a neurology practice, of course, a fair number of people with real brain tumors is to be expected. But they are rarely the same group seeking help primarily for their headaches. People with brain tumors are still a small number in the total practice of headache.

One of the most reassuring things that suggests that a patient doesn't have a brain tumor is the long-term presence of headaches that haven't substantially changed in character. Also, if the characteristic headache pattern is to feel perfectly well and from time to time get very sick with a headache, a brain tumor is unlikely.

When your doctor takes a medical history, certain facts about the nature of the pain and the symptoms that may accompany the pain are very helpful in diagnosing the kind of headache you suffer. If your headaches sound just like a migraine, a tension-type headache, or a cluster headache and your neurological examination is fine, you are likely to have the headache you describe.

Keeping a Headache History

When taking the medical history, your physician wants to know whether you have only one or more than one type of headache. How long the headaches have been present and whether they are changing is also important. A useful description of the headaches include the following: the first sign of an attack, how quickly it comes on, what symptoms accompany the headaches, how long they last, what triggers an attack, and what time of day or day of the week they occur. Your physician also needs to know how you are treating them at this time and how you have done so in the past. What were the results of those treatments, and what doses of medication were used in those treatments? How long did you persist with the suggested treatment? You should keep a headache history, recording these facts about each headache so you can report on patterns to your physician.

The single biggest obstacle in diagnosing headache type is the patient's inability to describe the attacks. It doesn't help to hear it's a "regular headache" and "you know everything else, after all, you are the doctor." The diagnosis of headache has to be a collaborative. *Frequent* and *severe* are subjective terms, and their meaning may be vastly different from person to person. A *bad headache* does not have a specific meaning to a physician.

The Neurological Examination

A neurological examination is complex and difficult for a layperson to understand. Most of the tests that are part of this examination seem silly, even fun for the patient. A physician will first test the ability to use language, organize tasks, and evaluate intellectual function and memory. Then he or she will assess the patient's mood. The medical history and the patient's responses obtain much of this information. Then the physician will examine the eyes with an ophthalmoscope, looking at the optic nerve and the surrounding blood vessels. The region of the eye viewed is actually an outpouching of the brain. For that reason, the evaluation with the ophthalmoscope gives an actual window into the brain. The pupils are examined and how they react to light, then how the eyes move when the patient gazes in different directions. The symmetry of the face and tongue and sensation to the face are checked. The physician might look into the throat and make you gag (this isn't fun). Then the muscles are examined to evaluate power and muscle tone. Reflexes are next, and it always surprises people that there are other reflexes besides those in the knees. Then the physician looks for disturbances in the sensory system by measuring pin or temperature sensation and the sense of position of joints, as well as the ability to detect vibration over joints. Coordination and how you walk are measured. The physician will check for tenderness over sinuses and whether those joints in front of your ears attached to the jaw are painful or clicking when you open your mouth. Arteries are examined for unusual sounds or tenderness, particularly in the neck and temples. The neck and shoulder muscles are noted to be relaxed or in spasm. You would be amazed how useful these simple tests are in determining who needs to proceed to further testing.

Headache Pattern and Brain Tumor

Having a migraine or cluster or tension-type headache doesn't grant you immunity to developing a brain tumor. Many neurology books describe a "brain tumor headache" as one that occurs in the morning and awakens you out of sleep. These get better as the day goes on but worsen over time. Most people with this history have perfectly benign headaches that are triggered by REM sleep. But if we hear this story, we pay extra attention.

Most people who develop brain tumors don't have this classic history. They usually note that whatever kind of headaches they used to get are getting worse; the headaches are more frequent and more severe. If you have migraine and are unfortunate enough to develop a brain tumor, you usually get more migraines as a manifestation of your tumor. If you have tension headaches and get a brain tumor, you'll get more of these. Remember that the brain is really not very sensitive to pain, so that headache is usually not a very prominent symptom of a brain tumor. Therefore it is important to be reevaluated by your doctor not just for a new kind of headache, but for worsening of an old kind. If there is a substantial change in the pattern of your headaches, you might need a scan of the brain.

Now before you get too anxious about all this, realize that when you have recurring headaches there will be good times and bad times, and that is natural. That seems to depend upon how many triggers you have encountered, and there are plenty of triggers that we can't easily identify. So only if the pattern is clearly changing over time is the reevaluation of your neurological status necessary.

Another common concern is that the headaches are going to lead to a stroke. They don't, although headaches can be one of many stroke symptoms. It is occasionally difficult to distinguish migraines from stroke. This confusion might occur when there is a migraine aura that causes one to lose speech, become paralyzed, or to develop numbness on one side of the body. In those special situations, a neurologist will generally do some tests aside from the usual. But almost always, when the symptoms indicate a migraine, it turns out to be a migraine. In Chapter 3 we talked about comorbidity. There are other conditions that are comorbid with migraine aside from psychological conditions. One of them is stroke. If you have migraine, you do have an increased chance of having a stroke or developing heart disease compared to those without migraine. It's not appropriate to worry about that too much since the increased risk of stroke when you have migraine is low. But it might be an additional incentive to do all the things you should be doing anyway, not smoking, losing weight, watching your cholesterol (not watching it go up), and exercising. That is the appropriate way you should react to the information that having migraine increases your risk of developing **atherosclerosis** (hardening of the arteries).

Other Secondary Headache Syndromes

There are some other serious conditions that cause headaches and require medical attention (see Table 4-1).

A 72-year-old woman developed headaches in the past month. They were located all over her head, and she described aching of her shoulders, neck, and head. It had become painful to brush her hair, and she noted tenderness over her temples. She felt "just awful" and even had some weight loss and a low-grade fever. She noted that when she chewed her jaw ached.

When someone over 50 years of age develops a new headache that is associated with tenderness of the scalp or tem-

Table 4-1   Headache Classification

Headache Type	Symptoms
Primary headache syndromes	
Migraine	May begin with a prodrome: depression, food cravings, euphoria, irritability, yawning, cold hands and feet. Sometimes auras: visual disturbances, numbness. Pain is pulsatile or aching, often one-sided, worsens with movement. Often associated with nausea, vomiting, light sensitivity, and sound sensitivity.
Tension	Bandlike pain on both sides of head, relieved by over-the counter medications and rest. Often associated with a specific stress or a prolonged neck posture.
Cluster	Usually recur frequently during periods of 2 weeks to 2 months. Agonizing pain builds quickly, eye on affected side reddens and runs, clear liquid discharges from nose. Often start during sleep. Alcohol is a potent trigger.
Secondary headache syndromes	
Brain tumor	Headaches become more frequent and more severe. Substantial change in headache pattern.
Temporal arteritis	Patients are usually over 50. Tenderness of scalp or temples, general achiness, chewing painful. Can lead to blindness.
Idiopathic intracranial hypertension	Patients are usually obese women with irregular periods. Pain aggravated by coughing, sneezing, and bowel movements. Swelling of optic nerves can cause vision loss.
Malignant hypertension	*Significant* headache caused by severe elevation in blood pressure
Subarachnoid hemorrhage	Sudden onset of intense pain, like an explosion in the head.
Meningitis	Generalized headache involving back of head, often stiff neck, usually fever.

ples, it needs attention. This could represent **temporal arteritis**, an inflammation of arteries, which if untreated can lead to blindness in one out of three people. Usually people with temporal arteritis feel achy all over and generally awful. Often the scalp hurts even more when they are out in the cold weather. It's amazing how tender the scalp can become with this condition, and hair brushing can become quite an ordeal. Often, chewing food causes even more pain in the jaw or in the tongue. A simple blood test, an ESR (erythrocyte sedimentation rate), is performed. An abnormal ESR is highly suggestive of temporal arteritis. If temporal arteritis is suspected, a biopsy of the artery in the temple is indicated.

A 22-year-old obese woman complained of headaches throughout her head over the past 6 weeks. Her periods had become irregular. She heard pounding noises in her head. The pain was worse in the morning when she arose and tended to get better as the day progressed, although there was some degree of pain throughout the day. Whenever she would cough, sneeze, or bear down to have a bowel movement, the pain worsened. Recently, she developed double vision.

There's another syndrome, called **pseudotumor cerebri** or **idiopathic intracranial hypertension**, that we see from time to time. Most people with this (but not all) are women, often overweight, and often with irregular periods. The description of these headaches resembles that of a brain tumor. Looking into the eyes with an ophthalmoscope, a swelling of the optic nerves called **papilledema**, is visible. A CTT or MRI scan will determine there isn't a tumor. Next is a spinal tap to measure the pressure of the spinal fluid (which is very high in this condition) and make sure there is no infection around the brain.

Usually medications are indicated to improve the headache and bring the spinal fluid pressure down. Aside from the headache, there is always the risk of vision loss with pseudotumor cerebri, so it is important to accurately diagnose this problem. Surgical treatments to reduce the pressure in the brain are occasionally needed. Managing this problem requires a collaborative effort between you, your neurologist, and your ophthalmologist.

Most headaches occur around the eye. Most people who seek help for headaches have already been checked out by their eye doctor who tells them everything is fine. How can that be?

The nerves that supply almost everything that is sensitive to pain within the head also supply pain sensation to the eye. Because they share a nerve supply, most pains emanating from the head (including migraine and cluster headaches) are felt above, below and deep inside the eye. This is called **referred pain**. It is the same phenomenon that can cause pain to radiate down the left arm with a heart attack. So, is it always necessary to see your eye doctor if your headache is centered around the eye? Not if you have had your headaches for a while, your eyes are not red, and your vision seems fine. The exceptions to this rule are rare, so let your doctor decide if you really need that appointment.

> *A 66-year-old man had a history of high blood pressure. When it was diagnosed, he had headaches that ceased when the blood pressure was treated a year ago. As he was feeling fine, he stopped his blood pressure medications. Since he had no return of his headaches, he felt satisfied that his blood pressure was fine.*

A common fallacy is that you get headaches from high blood pressure and that you can even predict your blood pressure from your headache. There are several problems with this. First of all, it isn't true. All but the most severe elevations of blood pressure aren't associated with headache. That means a lot of people aren't getting treated properly for increased blood pressure. The only way to know if your blood pressure is high is to have it taken. However, huge elevations in blood pressure, called **malignant hypertension**, can cause significant headache and are treated as a medical emergency.

A 48-year-old man noted that over the past 3 weeks, whenever he had an orgasm, he would develop a severe headache in the front of his head that came on over seconds. The pain would last several hours and was associated with some nausea and light sensitivity. He never had headaches like this before and was afraid to have sex.

There are countless jokes with the punch line being "not tonight honey, I have a headache." There is nothing funny about having headaches that come on with sexual activity. Sexually induced headaches are related to several other kinds of headaches that come on with exertion, including headaches that may arise from weightlifting or simply sneezing or coughing. Being at a high altitude seems to predispose to these headaches as well. Some people get fairly severe headaches at the time of orgasm. Sometimes these come on pretty quickly and are only too reminiscent of those that occur with a ruptured aneurysm of the brain. Most of the time these orgasmic headaches are benign, but should always be checked out since it is not impossible that you have ruptured a cerebral aneurysm during sex. They are disabling but ultimately disappear with treatment. Several medications are effective to prevent these attacks when taken prior to having sex. At other times, orgasm simply brings on a headache that is probably a tension headache and is usually easy to treat. The recent introduction of Viagra to treat impotence in men has increased the number of men complaining of headaches with sexual intercourse. Headache is the most common side effect of Viagra, probably because the drug can dilate arteries.

A 40-year-old woman came to the emergency room after experiencing the most severe headache she had ever had, which came on over seconds. She felt as if there was an explosion in her head. Although she was feeling better, her neck was stiff.

Among the most serious headaches we see are those due to a ruptured aneurysm within the brain. This is caused by the breakage of a weak area in the wall of an artery around the brain. There are other causes of bleeding of this sort, but they all result in what is termed a **subarachnoid hemorrhage.** Usually when a cerebral artery ruptures, it is unrelated to other headaches you have had in the past. The headaches of subarachnoid hemorrhage are strikingly abrupt in their onset. It's the worst headache you have ever had; it's like being shot in the head. This comes on over seconds, not minutes. If this ever happens to you, get to the emergency room of the closest hospital. They are going to do a CTT scan of your brain and possibly a spinal tap, which you might not like, but you should not bet your life that it will be normal and refuse the study. If blood is found in the spinal fluid, you will need other tests as well. Ruptured aneurysms in the brain aren't common, but they are nothing to ignore. Even if you feel better in a short while, or respond to some medication you take, the situation needs to be checked out fully.

For reasons never clear to me, nothing strikes more fear in

the heart of a headache sufferer than the mention of a spinal tap. Whenever a neurologist recommends a spinal tap be performed, friends and families all share with that patient a story they heard of someone who had one of these and then became paralyzed. Other friends always want to share their understanding that this is the most painful thing you can ever do to a human being. We will confess that spinal taps, like root canal, are not something you would independently solicit, but these tales of horror just aren't justified. Under local anesthetic the needle is placed well below the level where the spinal cord has ended, so no one can be paralyzed by this procedure. It just doesn't happen.

Spinal taps give us information we cannot obtain in other ways. We can measure the pressure of the spinal fluid, culture for bacteria and other organisms, and check for bleeding that might have been missed on a CTT scan (CTT scans detect most, but not all cases of subarachnoid hemorrhage). There is one other problem with getting a spinal tap. About 1 in 4 people get a spinal tap or **post-lumbar puncture headache**. Being thin seems to predispose some people to developing this complication. This headache is certainly unpleasant, but easily distinguished from most others. If you get a post-lumbar puncture headache, you note that when you are lying down it is gone. But it comes on again as soon as you stand up. It may be helpful to lie down for several hours after having a spinal tap and to drink a lot of liquids. It is a known complication of the test; it is not a sign that your doctor did anything wrong. Ultimately, it is going to go away no matter what you do, but if it isn't gone after a few days, you might consider getting an **epidural blood patch**. This is done by injecting a little of your own clotted blood into the site where you had the spinal tap; this commonly stops these headaches very quickly. Eventually, no matter what you do, post-lumbar puncture headaches go away.

Sinus disease, as already explained, doesn't often cause headache. This is not a hard and fast rule, and a CTT scan or other evaluation of the sinuses is sometimes appropriate.

Other infections, not only those of the sinuses, can cause headaches. In fact, an infection in any part of the body can cause headache simply through the mechanisms by which the body fights infections. Fever, itself, can cause headache. Some infections cause prominent headaches, such as Lyme disease, even if the infection itself is not in the nervous system. Among the most serious is an infection of the coverings of the brain and spinal cord called **meningitis**. There are many different organisms that can cause meningitis. Some are rapidly life threatening, others threatening over weeks and months; others, generally viruses, will go away without treatment.

The symptom of meningitis is a generalized headache that particularly involves the back of the head and can be associated with a stiff neck. Usually, but not always, you have a fever. The diagnosis is made with a spinal tap, and if your doctor suspects meningitis, there is no substitute for this test. Anyone with a headache, stiff neck, and fever should be seen by a physician on an emergency basis.

When appropriate, imaging tests are ordered. What are they? The CTT, or CAT scan, has been available much longer as a diagnostic tool, but it has not been entirely replaced by MRI scanning. For example, bleeding in the brain, such as occurs with a ruptured cerebral aneurysm, is much more readily detected with CTT than MRI. Assessing the sinuses is much better done with CTT. CTT scanning is also much faster, often accomplished in 5 minutes compared to 45 minutes or so with a MRI. Finally, CTT is much cheaper than MRI. However, evaluations of certain parts of the brain are best done with MRI. The spine at the level of the neck is better visualized with MRI, as is the back portion of the brain. No radiation is used when you get a MRI, in comparison to a CTT scan. At times, your doctor may order some contrast agent, administered into the vein in your arm, to enhance the scan. A dye containing iodine is used with CTT scan. The contrast agent used in MRI is an element with magnetic properties.

Electroencephalograms (EEGs) are not generally helpful in evaluating headaches, and their routine use for headache sufferers is not justified. However, there are exceptions to this. The same is true for thermograms. Psychological testing may be helpful in certain situations, but it is not routinely done, particularly if the headaches are not very frequent.

The history of the headache that you supply to the doctor, in addition to the neurological examination, is the best guide to determine whether any further testing is necessary.

5

What Causes Headaches?

It is important to remember that headache is just a symptom. It is not a disease. There are hundreds or thousands of possible causes of headache. However, diagnosis is usually not difficult because 90% of all chronic headaches are either migraine or tension-type.

Migraines

The cause of migraine is still elusive, but research has yielded a great deal of information in the last 15 years that has led to the development of some very effective treatments. Given the rate of research progress, we are likely to continue to see an explosion in the number of therapies to come in the next few years.

Migraine is very common. A large migraine study showed that 6% of men and 18% of women have this problem. For unclear reasons, these numbers may even be rising. Studies have also revealed that the prevalence of migraine rises each year, peaking at age 40, then begins to decline. This is good news if you are middle aged; it is likely that you will soon be better. It is bad news if you are a teenager. Women also assume that menopause is the reason they get better with old age. But it is clearly not that simple since men have their peak prevalence of migraine at the same age, although there are fewer men than women with migraine. It appears that migraine has a genetic basis and is inherited. If a parent has migraine there is a moderate chance that the child will have migraine. If both parents are migraineurs this probability is increased.

People with migraine are very prone to developing headaches in general. We don't have a better word than "headachy" to describe what is often a lifetime predilection to develop headaches. You may recall going to the beach with friends in the summer. Everyone else has a good time; you go home with a headache triggered by heat. Everyone has a wonderful time at a wine tasting. You awake with a headache in the middle of the night. Every time you get a fever, you get more headaches than your nonmigrainous counterparts with the same illness.

Migraine has been referred to for decades as a type of **vascular headache**. That's because we knew that vascular structures, or blood vessels, were involved. Most doctors learned in medical school the Wolff theory of migraine. Dr. Harold Wolff was the Chairman of Neurology at New York Hospital in the 1930s. Dr. Wolff theorized that migraine auras, when present, were caused by constriction (closing) of blood vessels, so you didn't get enough blood to the brain. The headache phase, it was said, followed when the blood vessels dilated, or enlarged. At this point one simply got too much blood to the brain, causing the arteries to become stretched and painful. There are quite a few bits of evidence to support this line of thinking. For example, at times you can actually see and feel stretched, dilated, and distended arteries in the temples during a migraine attack. People learn that if they put pressure over those arteries, they may feel somewhat better. Alcohol causes arteries to dilate, and if you have migraine you soon learn that drinking alcohol might trigger an attack of migraine. Heat also makes arteries dilate, and that's why a hot bath or a day at the beach can get you into trouble.

We now have a variety of sophisticated technological methods to measure blood flow in the head that were not available to Dr. Wolff. One of the problems with his theory is that there aren't any major changes in blood flow in brains of people who have migraine without aura. If you have migraine with aura, there are changes similar to what he predicted, but the timing of the changes in flow doesn't match when you get the aura or when you get the headache. So it seems clear that the changes he predicted are certainly not the whole story. The other problem is that that model didn't get us anywhere in developing effective treatments.

A lot of attention has been directed to the nerve supply of these blood vessels and discovering ways to alter their control of artery size and resulting blood flow. After all, arteries don't do much contracting and expanding on their own. Nerves controlled by the brain tell the arteries what to do. Nerves communicate with each other and the structures they supply by releasing chemicals at their ends. These chemicals are called **neurotransmitters**. A lot of neurotransmitters are already known, and different nerves release different neurotransmitters. After the neurotransmitters are released, they attach to a receiving station on the other side, called a **receptor**. More than one type of receptor may be able to receive a signal from the same neurotransmitter, and these different types of receptors may function differently. Different neurotransmitters and different receptors are present in different parts of the body. When these receptors receive the neurotransmitter that is released, they either turn on or turn off the structure on the other side.

There is a fundamental difference in the way that blood vessels in the head, as opposed to the rest of the body, receive their nerve supply. There are tracts of nerves to blood vessels that are important in supplying sensation to the head as well as making blood vessels alter their size. These nerves, called trigeminovascular neurons, are not seen in any other part of the body, and the chemistry of their neurotransmitters is also unique. Trigeminovascular neurons conduct the pain that we experience in migraine. But this doesn't tell us where the migraine attack actually begins.

It has always surprised people when we explain that the brain isn't very sensitive to pain and that structures outside the brain are involved in pain production. A classic example is the 1847 case of Phineas P. Gage, a railroad foreman, who set a blast too early and ended up with a $3\frac{1}{2}$-foot iron rod through his skull. It entered the left side of his face, fracturing his cheek bone, penetrating the floor of his left eye chamber, and slicing through the anterior (front) lobe of his left cerebral hemisphere. The rod exited, fracturing the parietal and frontal skull bones. A little bit of his brain was left coating the rod. He made a few convulsive movements but was conscious and talking after the injury. The next day he was delirious, but he recovered quickly and was left with scars and loss of sight in his left eye. Not once did he mention pain, and his mental faculties remained intact. No one would have been surprised if he had complained of head pain. He had seriously injured his brain, yet had no headache.

Most of the interest in the chemistry of migraine has focused on one particular neurotransmitter in the brain, **serotonin**, also known as **5-HT**. It has been known for some time that levels of this chemical fall during an attack. One investigator gave intravenous serotonin to people with migraine and found that this stopped the migraine but had too many side effects to be considered a practical treatment. We know that when nerves tell arteries to expand (dilate), serotonin is an important chemical neurotransmitter to communicate this message. The majority of blood vessels in this regard are located on the outside of the brain, rather than in the brain. The brain isn't very sensitive to pain, but these blood vessels are. When they expand, they stimulate nerves that carry pain-producing messages into the brain, which we interpret as the throbbing pain of migraine. During the same process, other chemicals are released that make these arteries inflamed and swollen. When they swell, the arteries may become rigid. When that occurs, they may become so stiff that they can no longer stretch with normal pulsations of blood. The pain of migraine is ordinarily pounding, but as the attack progresses, the pain may become more achy and less pounding for this reason.

We believe that the structure that actually generates a migraine is located in a deep portion of the brain, called the **brainstem**. Some medications used to treat migraine appear to affect that structure. However, sumatriptan, a highly effective antimigraine agent, doesn't appear to enter the brain, yet still treats the attack. Therefore, other mechanisms of treating attacks are possible, and we really don't know whether a drug must enter the brain in order to be effective.

Many of the migraine triggers may act by dilating blood vessels. Certainly many drugs and foods capable of bringing on a migraine do this. Wine, for example, contains several chemicals that enlarge vessels. Caffeine actually constricts these vessels, which is why it is added to so many headache remedies. However, with frequent use of caffeine, vessels begin to depend upon this chemical to maintain their tone. When we stop caffeine, or even just delay drinking it, vessels might enlarge, triggering an attack of migraine. The way your body rids itself of heat on a hot day is by enlarging blood vessels. That's also why a hot bath or a day at the beach can trigger an attack.

The **triptans**, the newest class of migraine drugs, are designed to stimulate serotonin receptors that inhibit the dilation of the arteries and reduce the inflammation that is produced when these nerves are activated. They also directly reduce these nerves' abilities to transmit the message of pain production in the brain. It sounds complicated, and it is. We now know that even though the master molecule is serotonin, there are nearly 20 receptors for serotonin, each of which has different functions. Returning to the original study using intravenous serotonin to stop migraines, the troublesome side effects occurred because all serotonin receptors were being affected. Most of these receptors are not involved in the production of migraine. We want new drugs to function only at serotonin receptors relevant to migraine. The way that it is accomplished is to design small differences into the original serotonin molecule, making it work on certain targeted receptors. These are really designer drugs in the best sense.

But it doesn't make sense to think that the brain isn't important in the production of a migraine. How about those prodromes of migraine with mood changes? How about the auras that are manifested by changes in the visual system of the brain? The brain is involved in generating migraines even though it isn't producing much of the pain.

The generator of the attack appears to be located in the lowest parts of the brain, in the brainstem. A region in that area, when electrically stimulated, can bring on a migraine. These particular nerves turn off during sleep, and we know that sleep can often terminate a migraine.

Tension-Type Headaches

All of this pertains to migraine. What about tension-type headaches, which are, after all, the most common type of headache? This is also a confusing issue. In medical school, we learned that these were called *tension headaches* because the muscles of the scalp and shoulders were tense. Then other doctors said that was all wrong. What was tense, they said, was the patient. So they thought these headaches were just *stress headaches*, and that seemed to imply, that we were talking about a **psychosomatic** (without a physical cause) headache that wasn't real. So all the experts got together to discuss this, and they coined a new term, *muscle contraction headache*. Unfortunately, a lot of headache sufferers didn't have contracted muscles at all. And if they did, they weren't necessarily more or less contracted when they had the headache. The amount of contraction didn't correlate with the severity of the headache. So all the experts got back together again and they produced the current term, **tension-type headaches**.

One trouble many physicians had, however, was distinguishing between these two types of headaches. Many patients said that their headaches often started out like a tension headache and wound up like a migraine. Others said that their headaches often started out like migraines and then wound up like tension headaches. It seems that often the distinction between these two headaches is blurred. Sometimes migraines aren't that painful, and sometimes tension headaches are associated with some light sensitivity and nausea. Surely there must be a relationship between these entities. As we continue to understand the chemistry of migraine and the chemistry of tension headaches, we find more similarities than differences.

The physiology of migraine is slowly being elaborated, but the physiology of tension-type headaches is still quite a mystery. If it is a variant of migraine, then perhaps the muscles become the target organs of the brainstorm, whereas in migraine the blood vessels are most affected.

Eye Problems

Too often, eyestrain is blamed for causing what are really migraines. Remember that most headaches involve the region of the eye, but that doesn't mean an eye problem. However, eyestrain does exist. Getting new glasses can be quite a trauma as our eyes and our brain try to adjust to the new lens. During this time, it's quite possible to expect an increase in headaches of all kinds. This effect should go away in a week or two. If it doesn't, go back to the eye doctor. There is nothing wrong with taking some time to accustom your eyes to the new prescription. Do this by using the new glasses for part of the day, going back to the old prescription the rest of the day, and very gradually switching over to the new prescription. Your brain has a memory for the old prescription as it is learning the new one.

The other situation where the eye doctor is needed comes when there is pain in an eye that is red and tearing, or when you don't have normal vision in the painful eye. Glaucoma and other serious eye problems can bring on a painful red eye, and treatment is an emergency.

Migraine auras often involve some visual changes lasting up to an hour. They are generally caused by problems in the brain, not the eye. Sometimes you realize that everything in the left side of your vision is missing, when you look at a face or a page. You should know that it likely will be the same if you close either eye, and therefore it is a problem in the visual field (in the brain) and not an eye problem. Doing this little test can be very helpful information for your doctor and may save you a lot of unnecessary tests.

Cluster Headaches

If you have been diagnosed with cluster headaches, you may note that with each attack, your eye gets red and tears. That is part of the syndrome of cluster headache and not an eye problem.

Cluster headaches are not just a variant of migraine, and although there are similarities, the two types are usually easily distinguished. Again, the physiology isn't entirely known, but it appears that cluster headaches start in the brain, like migraines, with significant effects on blood vessels.

Sinusitis

Chronic sinus disease doesn't commonly cause headaches that come and go, but this rule is not invariable. The reason we bring it up is that migraines and tension-type headaches often cause pain in the front of the head and face, so it is easy to call this sinusitis and not treat it properly. Most of the drugs on the shelves in drugstores that claim to treat sinus headaches are just simple painkillers with a decongestant or antihistamine added. Therefore, if they work, that doesn't mean you have sinusitis. Furthermore, if you have significant sinusitis that needs treatment, they won't likely be adequate. Certainly, if you get an infected-looking drainage from your nose or are running a fever with these, have your doctor check it out.

Temporomandibular Joint Disorder

If you are getting pain when you chew or yawn or if you clench or grind your teeth and have pain around your ear or temples, temporomandibular joint (TMJ) dysfunction can be your problem. The temporomandibular joint can dislocate if the muscles which hold it in place become imbalanced. A classic example would be someone chewing on a large piece of meat, then developing a sharp pain in these areas. If this problem occurs, try eating soft foods for a while and take aspirin or an over-the-counter anti-inflammatory medication for a few days. If the pain continues, you will need to have your dentist check this out. The actual source may not be in the joint itself, but you may need some dental management to relieve the pain. Occasionally, medications to reduce muscle spasm and relieve inflammation are used.

Temporal Arteritis

If you are over 50 with pain when you chew, it can be a symptom of a serious medical illness called temporal arteritis (which is discussed in Chapter 4). Your doctor should know about this symptom as well.

6

Don't Make
It Worse

In Chapter 7, we will talk about various medical treatments for headaches. There are other things that you can, and should, do for yourself to minimize the problem. Many people are doing the wrong things and making their headache problem worse. To manage your headaches better, you need to understand headache triggers.

You should realize that most triggers are additive to each other. When they occur together they may reduce your headache threshold sufficiently to actually bring on an attack. For example, eating hard cheese may not normally bring on an attack, but it might if you were otherwise stressed. Remember, few triggers are actually the *cause* of headache. If you don't have an underlying headache problem, that trigger may not matter. This should help you realize why a trigger might cause a headache on one occasion and not on another.

That's not to say that the management and identification of triggers is unimportant. It may well be that once you have the problem of migraine, whether you have a lot of migraines or just a few migraine attacks may depend on how many triggers you encounter.

Food Triggers

Before discussing food triggers, you have to make a promise. Don't put this book down and vow never to eat any of the foods mentioned. There are many people whose headaches are at times triggered by certain foods. Usually, they have already figured this out. If you haven't already connected eating certain foods to triggering an attack, those foods probably don't provoke your headaches and you don't have to be careful to avoid them.

A great number of foods have been implicated in triggering migraine. It is important to understand that when we talk about these food triggers we're not saying that you are allergic to these foods. Allergies imply some kind of immunologically mediated trigger. When foods trigger migraine, they generally do so by involving the pathways that we've discussed in regard to changing blood vessels and inflammation. You can't take allergy shots to rid yourself of migraine triggers.

One of the chemical triggers in food is **tyramine**, which is present in basically everything that is fermented. These foods include ripened hard cheeses, homemade breads, alcohol, herring, sauerkraut, sour cream, and yogurt. Soft cheeses don't seem to be a problem because they don't contain significant amounts of tyramine. Even in hard cheeses, there seem to be different amounts of tyramine within the cheese. If you have a wheel of cheese, for example, the outside of the cheese has a higher tyramine content than the inside.

The most potent food trigger is alcohol. Wines and liquors contain several chemicals that are likely to bring on migraines. We are not talking about hangovers or even necessarily over-drinking. Many people find that half a glass of red wine is sufficient at times to bring on a headache, often overnight during sleep. Every type of alcohol is a product of fermentation and contains tyramine. Therefore any kind of alcoholic drink that you may use can trigger a migraine. Red wine has been particularly blamed for headache, probably because of the greater amount of flavored phenols extracted from the grape skins during its preparation. Alcohol itself dilates blood vessels and is a powerful trigger. If you read wine labels you may see "May contain sulfites" on a label. You can be sure that these wines contain sulfites to keep the wine looking attractive and to keep red wine from turning brown. So, if you're sensitive to sulfites, you should avoid these drinks.

Sulfites used to be employed widely by food services. At home when you core an apple and leave it out for a while it turns brown. But, strangely enough, you could go into restaurants with open salad bars, and the apples, lettuce, and other vegetables would look great throughout the day. Their secret was to spray metabisulfite liberally on these foods, which prevented them from oxidizing. The FDA has outlawed this practice, but metabisulfites are still present in some products, for example, dried fruits, and some people with migraine are very sensitive to this. It is also present in certain pills. Some manufacturers, particularly of white pills, may put metabisulfites into their pills to keep them looking pretty.

Nitrites (known to cause blood vessels to swell) are added to cured meats to preserve their red color, as in ham, bacon, salami, and hot dogs. Some people are sensitive to them, giving rise to the name "hot-dog headaches."

The neurotransmitter **glutamate** in monosodium glutamate (MSG) has been associated with Chinese food and orig-
inally was listed as part of the **Chinese restaurant syndrome**.
Most people with headaches learned to look for restaurants
that said "no MSG" on their windows and menus. However,
MSG is used in high concentrations in soy sauce and other
sauces that are used in Chinese food. So even if they didn't
add MSG powder, there is plenty of it in the food. Despite this,
don't spend all your time blaming Chinese restaurants for triggering your headaches, even if MSG is a trigger. Lots of pre-
pared foods have plenty of MSG, for example, frozen foods and
potato chips. You should also be aware that *hydrolyzed food
protein, natural food flavoring, hydrolyzed vegetable protein*, and
other terms are perfectly acceptable as a substitute term for
MSG. So food labels may deceive you into thinking that there
is no MSG, when there is plenty in these products.

Other assorted foods that have been implicated as migraine
triggers include nuts, citrus fruits, bananas, chicken liver and
paté, broad beans, fava beans, and lima beans.

Many widely used foods contain caffeine. Coffee is a particularly common supplier of caffeine, and many people drink
it in large quantities. You may argue, "Then how come so many
headache medications contain caffeine?" The answer is that caffeine is a mild constrictor of arteries and the pharmaceutical
industry realized years ago that adding some caffeine to whatever else they were using can help headaches. You should realize that if you drink a lot of caffeine, however, you may begin withdrawing between doses and this withdrawal can
become the trigger of your next migraine. This is one reason,
although not the entire explanation, why some people have
headaches if they sleep too late. If you drink a lot of caffeine
in the mornings and on the weekends you sleep late and de-

lay your intake of caffeine, that can trigger a headache. Varying your awakening time can also precipitate a headache through a different mechanism. If you drink a large amount of coffee, you should consider reducing it, but you should do it gradually. If you attempt this quickly, you'll simply develop withdrawal effects and trigger more headaches and you'll give up this whole project quickly. Also, be aware that caffeine as well as several chemicals that are closely related to caffeine can be present in other foods, including many soft drinks, not just colas. It is also present in a number of pills that you might take for your headaches, such as Excedrin Migraine™, leading to an increased chance that those products can lead to rebound headaches.

The chocolate story is also complex. Many headache sufferers are convinced that chocolate triggers their headaches. For some that might be true. We are familiar with food preferences and food aversions as part of pregnancy, like a woman suddenly eating ice cream daily when she never liked it before. This has a neurological basis. The same is probably true of chocolate. We think that a craving for chocolate can be a symptom of a migraine prodrome. Therefore, if the earliest symptom of a migraine is a craving for chocolate and you act upon it, you might conclude that the chocolate triggered the migraine. But that might not be the case, and you may have suffered a migraine whether you ate chocolate or not.

Ice cream eating doesn't trigger migraines, but may trigger a distinctive headache in some. This can be a fairly intense ache in the front of the head that resolves when your palate thaws out. The cause is the cooling of nerve structures in the back of the throat. It has nothing to do with chemicals in the ice cream. The best treatment is not to eat ice cream. Frozen yogurt is no better.

In general, dietary triggers of migraine probably precipitate headache only in combination with other factors. That is why each case is individual. For example, you might have to eat chocolate at a certain time in your menstrual cycle and be stressed at the same time to experience a headache. When foods trigger migraines, they do so shortly after eating them. So don't worry about what you ate two days ago.

Fasting is also blamed for causing headaches, but studies show that headache with fasting does not necessarily mean you have low blood sugar. The trigger can be a relative drop, even if your sugar remains in the normal range.

Other Headache Triggers

All headache triggers are not foods. Stress is a very powerful trigger of migraine. You have only to watch television to realize that viewing something stressful may be followed very quickly by a migraine. In studies of real-world situations, we find that the relaxation following stress is a more powerful trigger. Many people actually find that stress is protective and that while they are stressed they're better, but as soon as they relax they feel worse. This is one of several reasons that migraineurs do so poorly on weekends and vacations. Who said, after all, that life is fair? The mechanism probably has to do with peak levels of stress and background excitation, which is discussed more fully in Chapter 4.

Sleep can both trigger a migraine and terminate a migraine. Particularly with children, a short nap often stops a migraine and should be encouraged. The sleep stage called REM (rapid eye movement) sleep is when you dream. REM sleep is a very powerful trigger of migraine. Most of your REM sleep occurs in the early morning. If you wake at 4 A.M. with a migraine and then go back to sleep, you will often find that you will spend a great deal of time dreaming, only to awaken shortly thereafter with a worse headache. These headaches often persist throughout the day and are very hard to deal with. Therefore it becomes important to treat a headache when awakening, not just to go back to sleep hoping it will disappear. Since time does matter when it comes to abortive medications, you need to be aware that you are usually quite behind in treating that headache by the time you awaken with it. You may resist getting up, but the only way to rid yourself of the headache is to get out of bed and take your abortive medication before going back to sleep. When you oversleep, you are also fasting, and that also may play a role in these "oversleeping headaches."

We also know that many migrainous women experience worse attacks just before or at the beginning of their periods. This is because of estrogen withdrawal. We'll talk about this later, but understanding this mechanism has implications for the way we treat not only **menstrual migraine**, but also how we treat migraine in women undergoing estrogen replacement therapy when headaches persist during and after menopause.

What happens if you take birth control pills? Most birth control pills contain a mixture of synthetic estrogens and synthetic progesterones, taken 21 days each month. Interestingly, if you have migraine and then take birth control pills, the migraines usually change. They may get worse, but they may also improve. If they worsen on one pill, they might not worsen on another. If you can't take any estrogen-containing birth control pill without worsening your migraine, a progestin-only tablet might be acceptable. Is it safe to take birth control pills if you have migraine? This has been argued for a long time, but it appears that it probably doesn't increase your risk of stroke significantly, with today's oral contraceptive formulations. As mentioned, there is some increased risk in having a stroke if you have migraine, but adding birth control pills won't substantially increase that risk. However, if you are a cigarette smoker and have auras with your migraines, there is a greater risk of stroke and it would be wise not to use birth control pills.

Odors, including perfumes and aftershave lotions, can certainly trigger migraines. Automobile exhaust can trigger attacks as well. By instinct, people with migraine appreciate a well-ventilated environment. There are so many reasons not to smoke, you shouldn't need another. But smoking can trigger headaches, and this includes exposure to someone else's smoke. Additionally, smoking increases the likelihood that you will develop hardening of the arteries and elevates your risk of stroke and heart attack.

Many medications can trigger headaches as a side effect, particularly if you are predisposed to headaches. If there is a change in your headaches, consider whether you have had a new medication introduced during that time period or whether there has been a change in the dosage of a medication you are already taking. The list of medications capable of inducing headaches is endless. For some medications this is a common side effect, including some drugs used to treat high blood pressure and some antidepressants. Since every clinical trial of every medication invariably includes someone who reports headache, simply finding it listed as a possible side effect of a medication can be deceptive.

Head injuries can be a powerful trigger of migraine. It is unclear how this happens. It is uncommon for headaches caused by head injuries to persist for years. When they go on forever, it is likely that you had an underlying headache problem before the accident.

Another trigger of headache can be changes in barometric pressure. I've seen people keep years of records of barometer changes and how it related to their headaches. It always reminds me of the quote from Mark Twain that "everyone complains about the weather, but no one does anything about it." If it is an important trigger for you, it's worth your while to anticipate this. Going out in the intense cold or coming inside after being exposed to cold can also be a problem.

High altitudes can trigger headaches, particularly if you exercise in that altitude. Try to spend several days in that area before doing strenuous exercise, if you are able. Occasionally, taking a diuretic, acetazolamide, for a few days and throughout that trip can help prevent altitude headaches.

Problems with Medications

After you have studied triggers, however, you have to accept the fact that no matter how carefully you manage your triggers, you are still going to get some migraines. Therefore as the only treatment of migraines, trigger management is almost never fully satisfactory.

Ideally, we would like to treat everyone without medications, since every medication has its share of side effects and risks. It was shown in 1992 that almost everyone with headache is taking drugs. Only 5% of men and 3% of women were taking no medications. Among the remainder, most are taking over-the-counter medications, which aren't likely to be effective treatments. This probably reflects the fact that most people with migraine don't know they have migraine and certainly don't know that there are some good treatment options available. If you poll people with headache, three-quarters of those taking prescription medications are satisfied with them, but this is not at all true of those taking the over-the-counter (OTC) drugs.

A great many people with recurrent headaches end up taking medications very frequently to relieve their headaches. There are a variety of reasons for this. First is a fear of getting a bad headache and the desire to prevent it. It is easy to observe the truth that the longer you wait to treat a headache, the more resistant it becomes to later treatment. That seems all right, but often it is tempting to take pills quickly because "I can't afford to get a headache today." It is frequently difficult to predict the intensity of a headache early on. Sometimes, an attack seems to be innocuous but soon becomes miserable. Other times, a headache may seem to be a big problem at the start, only to diminish to nothing as the day progressed.

Rebound Headaches

We think that the early treatment approach is helpful unless the frequency of attacks is so high that you are taking these medications more than two or three times a week to treat headaches. The problem arises when you take medications too frequently, leading to **drug-induced** or **rebound headache**. That situation occurs when the next headache is caused by a withdrawal reaction to the last medication you took. The more medication you take, over time, the worse it gets. A transformation occurs, and what used to be an intermittent headache turns into a disaster called "chronic daily headache." Whatever drug you used that caused this syndrome will also become less effective over time. Let's say you start out with 10 codeine-containing prescriptions each week, then need 20, then 30, and so on. The more you take, the worse the whole problem gets.

Not all medications appear to induce rebounding under usual circumstances. That's the good news. The "triptans," dihydroergotamine, or the nonsteroidal anti-inflammatory medications have a low likelihood of inducing rebounding. However, even these drugs can induce headaches if taken very frequently. Using them two or three times a week is not likely to cause rebound.

The bad news is that the rebounding condition is progressive. The more medication you take, the more you need, and your headaches get further out of control. Furthermore, preventive medications don't work when you are in this bind, so your doctor can't give you some medicine that will make it all go away. It becomes no simple matter to stop the offending drug.

When you see your doctor, you are likely to be told that you must stop these drugs. My experience is that many are willing to try, but what happens with rebound headaches is that they get much worse before they get better. Many react to this experience with the comment that the doctor is crazy: "I told him I needed the medication." If you persist and don't restart the medication, often, after weeks, the headaches abate. On the other hand, if you don't stop the offending drug, it is highly unlikely that you will ever improve, and most likely your problem will gradually worsen and become even more difficult to manage. Clearly, prevention of this problem is easier than treatment.

Understand that we are not talking about addiction. This is a different syndrome, and rebounding seems to be a problem unique to headache sufferers. It's not clear why this is, but people with arthritis, for example, don't get rebound headaches from their pain medications, often the same ones that cause rebound headaches in migraineurs. It seems that this issue has to do with the unusual chemistry of the brain in someone with chronic headaches.

Sometimes people are so impaired from rebounding that they just can't manage at home. Other times, they are taking such large amounts of barbiturate or narcotic-containing medications that it's not even safe for them to treat themselves at home. Other times there is too much temptation for patients to restart the offending drug when it's available at home, which derails the detoxification process. In that setting, hospitalization becomes necessary.

Every headache doctor has had his or her own way of dealing with this problem. It was convincingly shown that an old drug, dihydroergotamine, is highly effective in treating rebounding. Patients feel better, allowing them to successfully stop everything that they were doing wrong. Unfortunately, this drug is too difficult to administer at home, even with home IV services, and is generally used in the hospital setting.

The following protocol is employed by most headache clinics in the United States. First, an evaluation by the primary doctor makes certain that there are no other medical problems that would make it unsafe to administer the drug, dihydroergotamine (DHE). These include heart disease, peripheral vascular disease, and high blood pressure that is not well controlled. We certainly would never use this medication in a pregnant patient. People are admitted to the hospital for 3 days or more. During that time the offending drugs are stopped, prophylactic medications are added, and the intravenous DHE is begun along with a medication to block the nausea that DHE commonly induces. During that hospitalization, we also bring in the physical therapists to teach the sufferer about triggers in the neck and how to relieve them. Stress management is taught.

Education is a major component of the treatment because getting better is a different process from staying better and patients tend to relapse into the same behaviors without this input. No one likes a hospital stay, but rebounding can be so severe that this step is necessary to successfully change the awful situation. Continuing to self-medicate will only make the situation worse as the brain becomes increasingly insensitive to treatment.

We can sometimes accomplish this on an outpatient basis. The use of repetitively administered triptans, such as Imitrex or Amerge, is currently being studied as a method of avoiding hospitalization while the patient withdraws from the offending medications.

7

What Can I Do About My Headaches?

When you understand that there is no such thing as a "regular headache," you can appreciate that there is no such thing as a generic headache treatment. What has advanced the treatment of headache is a better understanding of the processes in different kinds of headaches. Recognizing what is going wrong can lead us to develop treatments that interrupt or modify the pain pathways in different ways. We cannot cure most headaches yet, but we can manage them.

Certainly, the most exciting breakthroughs have come in the treatment of migraine. That's good, since this is the headache that generates the most complaints and has been notoriously difficult to treat.

It was shown several years ago that almost everyone who has migraine is taking some kind of pills. Most are taking over-the-counter (nonprescription) drugs; the rest are using prescription agents. The over-the-counter products are much less effective than the prescription drugs. The reason they are used so widely is that most people are treating themselves for headaches, rather than seeking medical care. This does not mean that nonprescription drugs have no value. The concern is that many people with migraine are still undertreated and could be managing their headaches better.

The first step is management of the triggers of headache, if you can identify them and limit them. Do not think that this will solve the whole problem, but trigger management may reduce the number of headaches you experience. However, you should always know your triggers and try to control them, even when you treat your headaches in other ways. It's important to understand that triggers provoke but are not the actual cause of the problem. No matter how well you manage your triggers, expect to reduce the number of headaches but not to eliminate them.

Natural Remedies

There were a number of reports that feverfew is a helpful natural treatment for migraine. In our experience, however, the efficacy of feverfew is minimal. A recent large study has also reported it to be fairly ineffective in treating headache. Feverfew can actually cause rebound headache. As with other natural treatments, the hope is to find some active ingredient that can be identified, then tested for safety and efficacy. Until that time, it is unclear whether this product is reasonable to use and even less clear that it is safe. In medical school we were taught that the definition of a drug without side effects is "one that is untested." The closer you look, the more likely there will be some untoward reactions to any product, natural or otherwise. Cyanide and strychnine are both natural, but poisonous. Natural and safe are not synonymous. That's not to say that natural remedies in headache management are value-less. It is just important to recognize that we never know as much as we should about either their safety or their efficacy.

Magnesium Supplements

Magnesium levels have been found to be low in red blood cells and in the brain tissue of some women with migraine at the time of their menstruation. Magnesium supplementation has been shown to be of benefit in the treatment of migraine, but probably for those women who have migraines a few days before their periods and suffer from PMS symptoms. Taking magnesium supplements daily, from the end of ovulation until the beginning of the period, appears to be of value in treating menstrual migraines in some women. It can cause diarrhea and is not always helpful.

Nonmedical Treatment of Headache

Physical therapy, chiropractic therapy, and massage therapy are all of value in the treatment of headaches, particularly with frequent attacks involving neck and shoulder pain, or when some movements of the neck seem to trigger a headache. The trigeminal nerves of the brain that we spoke about before are actually seen in the neck portion of the spinal cord. The first three nerves that exit the spine in the neck (named C_1–C_3) have connections to this system; therefore, it is not surprising that neck symptoms may accompany migraine as well as tension-type headaches. You have to understand, however, that this doesn't mean the actual cause of the headache is located in the neck.

Another treatment that may help is "sleep therapy." Sleep turns off the nerves in the brainstem that are turned on during a migraine. This seems to be a particularly useful treatment for children. If a child comes home from school sick with a migraine, an hour of sleep might just terminate the attack. It's useful in adults as well, but it is often more difficult for an adult to fall asleep with a migraine. If they do fall asleep, the benefits are less consistent. It seems that sleeping propped up with a few pillows, in a cool, dark, well-ventilated room is best. Most migraine sufferers know this by instinct.

You have probably noticed that if you have a migraine, concentrating on it too much will make it worse. If we pay particular attention to pain, it will always become worse. That's why every pain seems greater while lying in bed at night. Distraction often helps make the headache go away. Falling asleep, even "TV therapy" is useful, in addition to whatever else you are doing to treat a headache attack.

Exercise is always helpful when you have chronic pain. It is often quoted that you get relief through the body's production of **endorphins**, which are natural opium-like, painkilling chemicals your body produces, but there are lots of other explanations and benefits. If there is tightness of the neck, swimming, massage, and even rotations of the neck that you can do in the shower, can be beneficial. Try to avoid extreme movement and concentrate on gentle, low-impact exercises. Don't try to progress too quickly with your exercise program. You have plenty of time to achieve your goal once you are committed and begin your exercise plan.

There are a variety of devices on the market that are designed to either warm or cool the back of the neck. These can be helpful and worth trying at different temperatures in different attacks, although cold is usually favored. Resting in bed with a cold pack on the back of the neck, or around the temples and forehead, is reasonable. Sometimes the way you sleep, particularly the pillow you use, can affect headaches in the neck region. There are countless "cervical pillows" on the market and everyone has a favorite, so be willing to look around and experiment with these. It is amazing how intolerant we are to a change in our pillows. A new pillow can be a problem. You might consider bringing your own pillow from home when you travel.

Abortive Medication for Migraine

In discussing medications to treat migraines, it is best to divide them into groups. The first are **abortive agents**, drugs used to stop a migraine that has already started.

Our goal of treatment is to limit the migraine attack and its disability. We have been doing trials of migraine drugs for 22 years, and only recently have the goals of treatment shifted from simply pain relief to relief of **migraine disability**. This is not a trivial distinction. If we were testing a drug to relieve the pain of a broken arm, pain relief would be the goal. In contrast, remember that migraine is a "sick headache" and that lots of symptoms are present in the attack aside from pain. If we simply use morphine as the migraine treatment and give the patient a big dose, then ask him how much pain he has, he might reply, "not much," if he were awake. At the same time, he would likely be nauseated, sleepy, and certainly unable to return to work or play, even if the migraine pain were relieved. In that sense we have not treated the migraine disability. With many of the newer antimigraine drugs, migraine disability, with all of its components, is relieved. Migraine treatment is not optimal when you get only pain relief but you can't go on with your life because of drug side effects or nonpainful migraine symptoms, such as nausea, vomiting, and light or sound sensitivity.

Simple, over-the-counter pain medications are used widely by headache sufferers to get relief. These are generally used as self-treatment rather than having been prescribed by a physician. The major problem with this group is that these drugs are not very effective, or effective for only mild headaches. The advantage is that they are cheap and easy to take, and certainly readily available. You don't need a prescription. But they aren't free of problems either. They may cause rebound headaches, and if you take them too often they can lead to kidney and liver problems. Aspirin, if taken to excess, can cause stomach ulcers. It is never appropriate to give aspirin to a young child, for fear of developing a very serious disorder known as Reye's syndrome.

One class of medications used is nonsteroidal anti-inflammatory drugs (NSAIDs), which include ibuprofen and naproxen. These are generally prescribed, but several are now available over-the-counter without a prescription. Aspirin is also a nonsteroidal, anti-inflammatory medication, but acetaminophen is not. When they work, their advantage is that they don't make you tired and generally don't add to your nausea. It seems that NSAIDs, when used to treat headache, work best at high doses, even higher than is generally prescribed for arthritis. High doses result in greater side effects; so we are particularly concerned about the state of the kidneys and liver as well as the risk of developing a bleeding ulcer with the frequent use of these drugs. The over-the-counter doses of these drugs are often too low to stop a migraine. However, before taking big doses on your own, remember that when doctors prescribe these, they monitor the blood, which you can't do on your own.

Narcotics are used frequently to treat migraines. Examples include codeine, Percodan, Lortabs, and Stadol (see Table 7-1). They are rarely agents of choice, however. They are not very effective, often increase nausea, and certainly can lead to both addiction and rebound headache if used frequently. Just as important, they leave you tired and unable to function. That is not relief of the migraine disability.

Among prescription drugs, there are several products on the market that are similar and contain aspirin or acetaminophen with a barbiturate butalbital (Fiorinal, Fioricet, Esgic, Phrenilin, etc.). These are widely used to treat migraine, but are actually marketed to treat tension-type headaches. They are modestly effective. Advantages include reasonable pricing and general safety. They don't work by constricting arteries and will not increase the risk of heart attack if you have significant known or undiscovered coronary artery disease. The problems are that they will make you tired, generally work only for mild to moderate attacks, and if taken too often can lead to rebound headaches. It is hard to say how much is too much, but it is clear that they should never be used more than two or three times a week and should be restricted to fewer than ten tablets weekly.

Ergotamine tartrate (Cafergot, Wigraine, etc.) has been used for over 50 years to treat migraine. It is a powerful constrictor of arteries. Its use arose out of the understanding that migraine pain was due to enlargement of arteries in the brain, therefore the treatment should be to constrict them. However, our understanding of migraine has changed, and that mechanism is no longer the primary goal of treatment. An advantage of this drug is its effectiveness in treating migraine, especially if taken very early in an attack. A disadvantage is that it needs to be taken quickly. Frequent use can lead to rebounding, and it may take only a dose every week or two to create that situ-

Table 7-1   Medications for Headache

Medication	Form, Effectiveness, Side Effects
ABORTIVE AGENTS FOR TENSION-TYPE nonsteroidal anti-inflammatories (ibuprofen, naproxen, ketorolac, indomethacin, aspirin)	Effective for episodic headaches. Tablets available over the counter. Side effects with frequent use include kidney and liver damage and bleeding ulcers.
combination analgesics with butalbital (Fiorinal, Fioricet, Esgic, Phrenilin)	Effective for episodic headaches. Tablets. Side effects include sedation, rebound headaches with frequent use. Most contain caffeine.
PROPHYLACTIC AGENTS FOR TENSION-TYPE selective serotonin reuptake inhibitors (Prozac, Paxil, Zoloft, Celexa)	Possibly effective to reduce frequency of chronic headaches. Tablets. Side effects include insomnia, weight gain.
tricyclic antidepressants (amitriptyline, nortriptyline, doxepin)	Effective to reduce frequency of chronic headaches when taken preventively on a regular basis. Side effects include weight gain, dry mouth, sedation, constipation.
ABORTIVE AGENTS FOR CLUSTER oxygen	Often effective for cluster, though not other headache types. Breathed through mask from portable tank. No side effects.
sumatriptan (Imitrex)	Very effective by injection. Other forms of sumatriptan are not indicated. Can constrict coronary arteries so it is not used if an excessive risk of coronary artery disease exists.

Medication	Form, Effectiveness, Side Effects
PROPHYLACTIC AGENTS FOR CLUSTER	
lithium carbonate	Effective in reducing number of cluster headaches. Tablets. Side effects include thirst, frequent urination, tremor.
divalproex sodium (Depakote)	Effective in reducing number of cluster headaches. Tablets. Side effects include weight gain, hair thinning, gastrointestinal distress.
verapamil	Effective in reducing number of cluster headaches. Tablets. Side effects include constipation, lowered blood pressure.
corticosteroids (Medrol, prednisone, etc.)	Very effective in reducing number of cluster headaches. Tablets. Side effects include ulcers, bone loss, insomnia, weight gain.
ABORTIVE AGENTS FOR MIGRAINE	
nonsteroidal anti-inflammatories (ibuprofen, ketorolac, indomethacin)	Sometimes effective, but over the counter doses often too low to be effective. Tablets. Kidney and liver damage and bleeding ulcers are side effects with frequent use.
Cox II inhibitors (Vioxx, Celebrex)	Sometimes effective. Tablets. Fewer gastrointestinal side effects than other anti-inflammatories.
narcotics (codeine, meperidine, hydromorphone, propoxyphene)	Modestly effective. Tablet, injection, suppositories, nasal spray. Addictive. Side effects include sedation, nausea and rebound headaches.
combination analgesics with butalbital (Fiorinal, Fioricet, Esgic, Phrenilin)	Modestly effective. Tablets. Side effects include sedation and rebound headaches.

(Continued)

Table 7-1   (*Continued*)

Medication	Form, Effectiveness, Side Effects
Ergot derivatives	
ergotamine tartrate (Cafergot, Wigraine)	Effective when taken early. Tablets and suppositories. Side effects include nausea, rebound headaches. Also constricts arteries.
dihydroergotamine (Migranal)	Very effective. Nasal spray, injection. No rebound headache. Can constrict coronary arteries.
isometheptene (Midrin)	Modestly effective for migraine and tension-type headaches. Tablets. Fewer side effects than ergotamine tartrate. Side effects include rebound headaches and sedation. Might constrict coronary arteries.
Triptans	
sumatriptan (Imitrex)	Effective relief of all disabling migraine symptoms. Available as injection, nasal spray, and tablets. Nasal spray acts fast, has unpleasant taste. Injections not effective for headache if used during aura. All triptans can constrict coronary arteries. Side effects of triptans include flushing, and neck, chest, and jaw tightness.
zolmitriptan (Zomig)	Effective relief of all disabling migraine symptoms. Tablets. Can constrict coronary arteries. Can cause sedation as well as flushing and neck, chest, and jaw tightness.
rizatriptan (Maxalt)	Effective relief of all disabling migraine symptoms. Tablets and rapidly dissolving wafer that doesn't require water. Can constrict coronary arteries. Can cause flushing and neck, chest, jaw tightness, and sedation.

Medication	Form, Effectiveness, Side Effects
naratriptan (Amerge)	Slightly less effective than other triptans. Tablets. Lasts longer in the blood than other triptans. Can constrict coronary arteries. Well tolerated, fewer side effects than other triptans.
ADJUNCTIVE MEDICATIONS FOR MIGRAINE antinauseants	Effective for nausea associated with migraine. Available as tablets, injection, and suppository. Usually a sedative effect. Restlessness also a side effect.
PROPHYLACTIC AGENTS FOR MIGRAINE beta blockers (propranolol, nadolol, atenolol, timolol, metoprolol)	May take weeks to become effective. Side effects include fatigue, low blood pressure, depression, impotence, and exercise intolerance.
calcium channel blockers (verapamil)	Somewhat effective for lowering migraine requency. Side effects include constipation, male infertility, low blood pressure.
nonsteroidal anti-inflammatories (ibuprofen, naproxen, ketorolac, indomethacin)	Somewhat effective in preventing menstrual migraine when used just prior to predicted migraine.
Cox II inhibitors (Celebrex, Vioxx)	Somewhat effective in preventing menstrual migraine when used just prior to predicted migraine. Fewer gastro-intestinal side effects than other anti-inflammatories.
triptans (sumatriptan, naratriptan)	Effective in preventing menstrual migraine when used just prior to predicted migraine.

(Continued)

Table 7-1 (*Continued*)

Medication	Form, Effectiveness, Side Effects
ergots (methysergide (Sansert))	Modestly effective. Side effects include serious scarring around kidneys, heart, and lungs with prolonged use.
antihistamine (Periactin)	Reduces frequency of migraine, especially in children. Considered safe. Side effects: weight gain and sedation.
tricyclic antidepressants (amitriptyline, nortriptyline doxepin)	Low doses reduce frequency of migraines. Can be combined with beta blockers.
monoamine oxidase inhibitors (MAOI)	Somewhat effective, used only when other medications fail. Cause serious increases in blood pressure when combined with many foods or other medications.
selective serotonin reuptake inhibitors (Prozac, Paxil, Zoloft, Celexa)	Antidepressants with fewer side effects than tricyclics. Probably not effective for migraine. Effective for daily headache syndromes. Headache is a side effect that is minimized by starting with low doses. Side effects include insomnia and weight gain.
Anti-epilepsy drugs divalproex sodium (Depakote and Depakote ER)	Effective preventative of migraines and some chronic daily headaches. Tablets. Can cause weight gain, hair thinning, and gastrointestinal distress.
gabapentin (Neurontin)	Possibly effective in reducing migraine frequency at higher doses. Tablets. Side effects include sedation and weight gain.

ation. Unfortunately, the package inserts recommend more frequent use than is probably safe. Another problem with ergotamine is that it may cause nausea. Aside from the fact you don't want any drug to make you nauseated, it has been shown that drugs causing nausea are not likely to eradicate a headache. In the same way, narcotics make the headache worse when they make you nauseated and certainly if you vomit. If you have an aura, that is a good time to administer ergotamine drug. It won't help to shorten the aura, but the medication will be in the bloodstream to help get rid of the headache.

Most headache experts use ergotamine tartrate less and less each year as we have newer medications that are more specific for migraine. However, one of the old ergots is being used increasingly. This is called dihydroergotamine (DHE), which is a cousin of ergotamine tartrate with some significant differences. DHE has been available for years. It seemed to be a weak constrictor, so why use it when we had a stronger one like ergotamine tartrate? As the theory of migraine changed, we became interested in drugs that might alter some of the serotonin receptors. DHE was discovered to affect these receptors and proved to be safer and more effective than its cousin. Available only by injection, for years it was used primarily by headache experts when treating migraines in the emergency room and by a few souls motivated to give themselves a shot in their muscles to rid themselves of migraine. Recently, DHE was released as a nasal spray (Migranal) and is now easy to take at home. You have to use a gizmo where you break a glass vial, then snap a plastic sprayer over that. After priming it, you spray into each nostril, then repeat the dose in 15 minutes. Side effects are usually minor, and the drug often works quite well. If you have untreated high blood pressure or artery disease, including involvement of coronary arteries, you can't use this drug. The same is true if you are pregnant or breast feeding. Advantages include its effectiveness in moderate or severe attacks. Not only is it not likely to cause rebound headaches, it is actually used to treat rebounding.

A unique agent is isometheptene, which is combined with other ingredients as Midrin. This agent acts in many ways like a weak ergotamine tartrate, less effective but with fewer side effects even though this drug is not an ergot derivative. It is marketed to treat tension-type headaches and migraines, but is unlikely to be an adequate treatment for a severe migraine. It is relatively inexpensive. Like other constrictors of arteries, it can lead to rebound headaches if taken too frequently.

One of the most exciting advances in abortive migraine treatment came with the introduction of sumatriptan (Imitrex) in 1993. We now have several related medications on the market, which we refer to as triptans. The triptans are highly effective and generally relieve migraines without inducing a lot of side effects. Triptans relieve all the symptoms that lead to migraine disability: pain, nausea, and sensitivity to light and sound. Sumatriptan lasts only a few hours in the blood, which is great in one way, since you are medicated for just a short time. However, some migraines are long lived, and you may find that the headache recurs perhaps half a day later. Usually any recurrences are easy to treat with a repeat dose, but recurrences do occur up to a third of the time. A recurrence is different from rebounding. Rebounding results when drug withdrawal actually triggers the next attack. Recurrence reflects the fact that the migraine may last longer than the drug lasts in the body.

Initially, Imitrex was introduced as an injection, but more recently has become available as tablets and as a nasal spray. The injectable form remains the most effective migraine therapy available today. However, it does require you to inject yourself using a clever little gadget, a prefilled syringe with a gun. It is also available as a prefilled syringe alone for those who are willing to directly inject themselves. It is recommended that you do the procedure in your doctor's office the first time so that any side effects you might experience can be assessed by the doctor. A small risk of serious side effects does exist. The beauty of using injectable Imitrex is that you can treat yourself anywhere with a product just as effective as anything an emergency room can administer. That's comforting given how mobile many of us are today.

For the whimpier among us, Imitrex nasal spray is often used first, since it is fast acting and has very few side effects. The one side effect that stands out is its bad taste. A few people will say that they got good headache relief but won't take it because it isn't tasty. At any rate, the taste problem is short lived. It can also be solved by leaning forward and spraying the medicine into the front third of the nose and breathing normally rather than trying to snort the medications deep into the nose. Taking mints or butterscotch candies when using the spray will also help. For those who don't like the idea of a nasal spray, there are still tablets of Imitrex. These are small and easy to swallow, but they won't work as quickly as the other two forms.

Since migrainous auras have been thought to have something to do with impaired blood flow to the brain and triptans all constrict arteries, an early study was performed looking at the safety of sumatriptan when taken during the aura. The results were curious. It turned out that the drug was safe to take during the aura. But when taken at that point, it did not prevent the headache from occurring. That has some practical applications. If you are using a triptan and have migraine with aura, wait until the aura resolves and the headache begins before taking the drug. These drugs never shortened or prolonged the aura anyway. Furthermore, migraine auras are not invariably followed by migraine headaches. So if you wait for the headache, you might not need medication if it does not materialize. However, those studies were done with injectable Imitrex, which works very quickly. Those who typically have severe migraines might begin tablets or nasal spray a few minutes into the aura.

A second triptan came on the market in early 1998—zolmitriptan, under the brand name Zomig. This is a tablet and also easy to take. It is very similar in side effects, safety, and efficacy to Imitrex tablets. It seems that some people who don't respond to one might respond to the other, so it is worth switching products if the first isn't satisfactory.

In July 1998, rizatriptan entered the market as Maxalt. Like the other triptans this is a highly effective medication to stop a migraine. It is available as a rapidly dissolving wafer (MLT) and as tablets. Its onset is rapid, and significant side effects are infrequent. The MLT form is not more effective than the tablet, but is easier to use because you don't need to take it with water. This may encourage patients to take it more quickly.

Another triptan also introduced in the late winter of 1998 is naratriptan, which is marketed as Amerge. This product lasts longer in the blood than the ones just mentioned. That means that the chance of headache recurrence is lower, although this product is somewhat less effective than Imitrex, Maxalt, and Zomig. Headache recurrence also seems more likely to occur if you wait a long time before you take a triptan or if the medication works somewhat, but not fully. In that setting, repeating the dose in 2 hours with Imitrex, Zomig, or Maxalt, and in 4 hours with Amerge, may get rid of whatever degree of headache is left and reduces the chance that the headache will recur. With early treatment you may actually use less medication to control your attacks and get better results.

We are not permitted to mix different triptans or different ergots within the same 24-hour period. This means that if you started treating a migraine with an Imitrex tablet, then felt you needed the injection because you were vomiting the pill, this would be acceptable. But the same injection would not be an option if you had taken a different triptan initially.

As a class, all triptans can constrict the arteries of the heart to some degree. This can lead to the most feared complication, heart attacks. Side effects of triptans are few, but occasionally someone complains about the triptan effects with a pressure in the chest or jaw. Almost always, this is a benign side effect that has nothing to do with blood flow to the heart. However, occasionally it is difficult to distinguish between the triptan effect of the drug versus constriction of the heart arteries by the drug. In that setting, it becomes important for your physician to perform appropriate tests to make certain that you do not have underlying coronary artery disease. This evaluation needs to be completed before you retry these drugs. Some patients have argued, when these questions arose, that they would be happy to skip the heart tests and not take the drugs. However, once the question of coronary artery disease has been raised, it is important to know whether you harbor this condition, not just whether you are willing to stop these drugs.

Basically, this is a concern in someone who already has bad coronary artery disease that hasn't been recognized. Risk factors for developing this problem include cigarette smoking (shame on you), diabetes, being overweight, high cholesterol levels, and high blood pressure. It is also prudent for your doctor to administer these medications in the office on the first occasion. With these precautions, these drugs are actually quite safe, and the risk of bad things happening to the heart are less that one per million doses, which might be about the same odds as winning the lottery and retiring. Should your doctor conclude that you shouldn't take a triptan, you must also avoid DHE, ergotamine tartrate, and every drug that can constrict arteries.

More triptans are coming in the next few years, and it will be interesting to see how they differ from one another. They all seem fairly safe, and the tablets are equally effective and widely used. You will probably see some that are amazingly safe but less effective and some that are long lasting but slower to work. Physicians will be assessing how fast the headaches come on, how quickly nausea appears, and how long the headache is expected to last when they select the best product for an individual.

Adjunctive Medication for Migraine

The second type of medication is **adjunctive medication**, used with the abortive agents to treat additional headache symptoms but not the headache itself. Examples are medications to dispel nausea or the anxiety that may be seen with the attack. Antinauseants can be helpful, but they usually won't be absorbed into the bloodstream if taken as a pill. Therefore you need to get an injection, or at least take a suppository. For some reason, all of the antinauseants on the market are sedating. Therefore, if you take these, it is unlikely you can go right back to functioning. Occasionally, the anxiety that can accompany a migraine is overwhelming, and giving some sedation can be helpful. It is not a good idea to take any of these medications very often, and they all make you tired.

One of the benefits of the new abortive migraine drugs, the triptans and dihydroergotamine, is that they tend to treat all of the symptoms of the migraine attack, so that adjunctive medications are usually not necessary. Therefore you won't have to worry about the sedation that is induced by the drugs used to treat nausea or anxiety.

Prophylactic Medication for Migraine

Prophylactic medications are used to prevent attacks from occurring in the first place. These are generally used only if the migraines are very frequent or if the migraines are very hard to treat when they actually occur. We are particularly interested in using prophylactic medications when the sufferer is using abortive agents that are likely to induce rebounding if taken too often. The headache frequency is somewhat less of a concern if the abortive agents that are used have a low likelihood of inducing rebounding. These include the triptans, DHE, or the nonsteroidal anti-inflammatory drugs. Prophylactic drugs are only moderately effective. For example, a drug like injectable Imitrex (sumatriptan) is effective close to 90% of the time. On the other hand, prophylactic medications are likely to cut the number of headaches only in half. One also has to consider the amount of drugs taken when you use prophylactic medication. This means dosing every day, day after day, before these agents will work. As with all drugs, these have side effects that you will have to endure. If you are taking prophylactic medications and doing well, it is reasonable to slowly taper off of them from time to time. At some point, the migraines may get better on their own, and you may no longer need these agents. Of course, the converse may be true as well, and you could need even higher doses at certain times or a change of drug.

However, there is some research to suggest that having migraines over time might increase the sensitivity of the brain and lead to the development of more migraines. In that sense, not treating migraines may increase the problem over time. This is what we call **kindling**, which provides a good argument for the use of prophylactic drugs in people with frequent attacks.

We are hopeful that we will soon have a better chemical model with which to design prophylactic migraine drugs, but that doesn't exist at this time. What seems clear, however, is that acutely administered drugs and preventive drugs work through different chemical pathways. That is why drugs that you take to treat a migraine attack usually don't work to prevent attacks, and drugs that you use for the prevention of migraines are valueless to stop an attack in progress. So don't confuse these two applications.

Although there are a lot of drugs that are used to reduce the number of migraines, very few are FDA approved for that purpose. This doesn't mean that we are experimenting on people. These drugs are all FDA approved, so they are available to us, but for various reasons, the manufacturer does not market them for this purpose. A few rules need to be remembered. Realistically, expect a prophylactic drug only to reduce the number of headaches. It is rare that these drugs make the whole problem go away. It may take weeks of use before you know how effective these agents are going to be for your headaches. Increasing the dose quickly can't accelerate this process very much, and side effects are more likely to occur if the dose is rapidly escalated. This slow time frame is a fact of brain chemistry and how these drugs regulate receptors in the brain. Therefore, it doesn't make sense to stop these drugs after just a week or so and then go back to your doctor to try another one. Please have patience. Another pitfall is not allowing sufficient time for a drug dosage to be increased, if you are able to tolerate more, before discarding it. You might find that with a particular dose, things really seem to fall into place. Please don't compare your dose to your friend's dose. There are large differences between us, not only in body size, but also in our ability to metabolize medications.

Probably the most commonly prescribed prophylactic antimigraine drugs are **beta-blockers**. Beta-blockers are a class of drugs that block receptors in the head called **beta adrenergic receptors**. There are a lot of these beta-blockers on the market, but they are not interchangable. Propranolol, nadolol, atenolol, and timolol are the ones that have antimigraine properties. Like all preventive drugs, it may take weeks for these drugs to become fully effective. Side effects include fatigue and depression; they may lower your blood pressure. Beta-blockers may also lead to impotence in men. As you might imagine, this class might be a good choice if you have high blood pressure and you also have migraine. If you have diabetes or asthma, you can't be on this class of drugs. Some people get a generalized feeling of weakness.

Although used widely, calcium channel blockers are only modestly effective in preventing migraines in most people. Among them, verapamil is the most likely one to work. These drugs also lower blood pressure and can be quite constipating. It has also been recognized that these drugs can induce infertility in men and, in fact, there are calcium channel blockers being studied as possible male birth control pills for the future. It is important to remember this side effect when a man is on these drugs and the couple wants a pregnancy. If you have both high blood pressure and migraine, it is particularly worthwhile to try this class of drugs.

The same nonsteroidal anti-inflammatory drugs that are used to stop a migraine may also have some value in preventing migraines. Generally, the time to consider them is in **menstrual migraine**. They work best in a situation where the attack is very predictable. Many women with menstrual migraine reliably have a migraine a day or two before their period, or just when the period begins. If their periods are regular enough, they might be able to pretreat the attacks with some of these agents and prevent the migraine. If you really don't know when the migraine might begin, this whole approach doesn't apply since you can't take these drugs in an open-ended fashion. Recently, impressive results have been reported using Amerge or Imitrex prophylactically for menstrual migraine as well.

Sometimes ergots are used preventively. One such product, methysergide (Sansert), has been marketed for years and works fairly well. We don't use this drug very often, however. It has been shown that serious scarring around the kidneys, heart, and lungs can occur, particularly with prolonged use. It is mandatory, if you are on methysergide, that you take a **drug holiday** periodically, which does minimize the likelihood of these problems developing. The drug holiday means that you must be off the drug for one full month after being on it for 4 to 6 months. It is important that you take this holiday very seriously. Some physicians have had the experience of having patients tell them that they were taking such a respite while they are secretly obtaining the drug from another physician. It is also important that, when you are taking your time off, you are not treating your breakthrough headaches with some other form of ergot, like ergotamine tartrate or dihydroergotamine. If you do, your drug holiday may not be valid and you might unknowingly risk the development of these serious medical complications.

There is a very old drug, cyproheptadine (Periactin), that is an antihistamine with antiserotonin effects as well, which has been used for decades to reduce migraines, particularly in children. It is said to be very safe and doesn't require a lot of blood tests to manage migraine. It is, however, fairly sedating and can lead to a lot of weight gain. Although always cited as very safe, the sedation issue is serious. Impairing a child's ability to think and remember is not benign.

Several drugs used to treat depression are also used to treat migraine, as well as tension-type headaches. Similar chemical problems occur in the brain with depression as in headache. Often, headaches respond to very low doses of antidepressants that would be too low to treat depression. Fortunately, when the doses are low, so is the rate of side effects. Remember that it is also common for headache patients to be depressed, in which case, the doses need to be adjusted accordingly. In that way you may "kill two birds with one stone." (We hope our parrot, Rodan, doesn't read this.) The antidepressants we use the most are called tricyclic antidepressants. They often have a lot of side effects including sleepiness, constipation, dry mouth, and weight gain. The fact that they are sedating is often a problem, but if you can't sleep at night or awaken too early in the morning with your headache, you might turn this into an advantage. However, we can often employ low doses, which minimize side effects. Certainly if you have migraine and are also depressed, the use of these drugs is logical.

Another class of antidepressants is called monoamine oxidase inhibitors (MAOI). These may work when other medications fail. The problem with these drugs is that they are potentially quite dangerous. Taking them with many foods, particularly those containing products of fermentation, can lead to serious or even fatal increases in blood pressure. Additionally, most of the medications that you might take for a bad headache cannot be used if you are taking MAOIs. Therefore, its use is largely restricted to situations where all other approaches have been exhausted. At the same time, you must be trained by a dietitian to avoid all the foods that interact with these drugs. You have to be compulsive about learning what ingredients are in foods that you did not prepare yourself.

A newer class of antidepressants, selective serotonin reuptake inhibitors, SSRIs (Prozac, Paxil, Zoloft, and Celexa), often have fewer side effects than the tricyclics. They are not as well studied as migraine drugs, and it isn't clear how useful they will be for migraine treatment. They are good choices for some of the daily headache syndromes. Unfortunately, one of the most common side effects we see is headache, but that usually settles down and can be minimized by starting with very low doses and raising them slowly. Sometimes these medications keep you awake. If you take them in the morning and they keep you awake, try taking them at night to readjust your biological clock. If you now take them at night and can't sleep, try switching to the morning. Many with migraine benefit from these medications for their symptoms of depression, even if they don't help the headaches. There is a very rare interaction between the SSRIs and the triptans referred to as a **serotonin syndrome**. This syndrome causes confusion, flushing, and twitching. The fact remains that millions of people have used these two classes of medications together without problems. If there is concern, administering these together in the doctor's office on the first occasion would be wise.

One drug that has been on the market for years to treat epilepsy, divalproex sodium (Depakote), is perhaps the most effective preventive antimigraine drug we have. The good news is that when you treat migraine, as opposed to epilepsy, with this drug relatively small doses are needed. That's good, because divalproex sodium can cause you to gain weight and not many are happy about that. Most of the time this doesn't happen, however, and being aware of this potential usually keeps people behaving themselves with an appropriate diet. It also occasionally causes hair thinning. It seems that your hair can become more brittle when you take divalproex sodium; taking vitamins with selenium and zinc and washing your hair with selenium-containing shampoos usually deals with this problem. It is rare that someone discontinues divalproex sodium for this side effect, which generally resolves over time on its own. Finally, the blood has to be monitored from time to time although blood abnormalities caused by this drug are very rare. This agent is clearly helpful in reducing the number of migraines and often helps some of those chronic daily headaches that are notoriously difficult to treat. Often it begins to work fairly quickly, although it tends to work even better over time. A newer form of Depakote, Depakote ER, has just been introduced to the market. This form has fewer side effects than Depakote, in particular less likelihood of weight gain.

You will see the use of other anti-epilepsy drugs in migraine treatment as well. The one gathering a lot of interest is **gabapentin (Neurontin)**, but there are too few studies out at this point to let us know how effective it is going to be. The beauty of gabapentin is its ability to avoid interactions with other drugs in the body and the fact that we don't need to check blood tests. Other anti-epileptic drugs will almost certainly be tested for any migraine preventive properties they may possess.

Estrogen Levels and Migraine

Treating migraine in women has additional challenges since migraines are often influenced by hormonal factors. Among young children, boys are more likely to have migraine than girls. Girls soon catch up and pass the boys in developing migraine at puberty. This is the first bit of evidence that hormones are involved with the development of migraine. When women get pregnant, their migraines are very likely to go away, at least in the second and third trimesters of pregnancy. For women taking birth control pills, headaches often worsen. Women are most likely to have a migraine problem in their early 40s, and this tends to improve after menopause. So it seems that hormones, and in particular, estrogen, are an important influencing factor for migraine. The major way estrogen influences migraine is to trigger an attack when the levels of estrogens fall. We call these **estrogen withdrawal headaches**. This is what happens before the period begins, although the actual menstruation is an effect of the withdrawal of progesterone and not estrogen.

When migraine occurs with the period (menstrual migraine), it is notoriously difficult to treat. The principles and medications used in treating this are the same as in all migraine, although there are a few additional tricks. Some women do better if they take a nonsteroidal anti-inflammatory medication daily for a few days before the period (or the expected time of the headache). If you are on a prophylactic medication that works pretty well except around the time of the period, transiently raising the dose before the period begins might help. Occasionally, we add estrogen patches before the period to blunt the fall in estrogen levels triggering the headache. Magnesium, discussed elsewhere, can also help. Diuretics (water pills) have been used widely. They reduce the bloating you might get with your period, but don't do very much to reduce the headache. As mentioned earlier, prophylactic triptans seem to be very effective in reducing menstrual migraines.

A lot of women are perfectly willing to have a hysterectomy in order to rid themselves of headaches. This is usually a big mistake. First, it's not the menstrual period per se, but the estrogen effect that is the problem. The ovaries make estrogen, not the uterus, so removing it does not make any sense. The problem is that if the ovaries are producing their own estrogen, even if we give estrogen medications, there still may be rising and falling levels that can trigger an attack of migraine. If we are desperate and convinced that estrogen withdrawal is the problem; we can always bring on menopause through drugs called GnRH analogs, although this type of chemically induced menopause is reversible when the drug is discontinued. We can then regain control of the estrogen level, not allowing it to fall, by using long-acting estrogen preparations. None of this is done often, and most of the time the migraines are treated by more conventional methods.

A 52-year-old woman had a long history of migraine with her periods. They were difficult to treat. She was delighted that after menopause last year, they went away. Wanting to have estrogen replacement therapy, she was placed on Premarin. Now her migraines are back, and she doesn't know what to do.

After menopause, the levels of estrogen are low and estrogen withdrawal is not a big issue. Frequently, when a woman who had migraines that were severe around her periods becomes menopausal, the whole problem goes away. Then she starts taking estrogen replacement therapy (ERT), and the headaches come back. Whether it is good or bad for you to take estrogens after menopause is controversial, and we are not going to discuss all of the arguments. Certainly estrogen replacement therapy helps retard the development of coronary

artery disease and also reduces the risk of developing osteo-
porosis. Is it possible to have it both ways; take estrogen and
still benefit from a natural reduction of migraine that being
postmenopausal brings? The answer is maybe.

You can't predict what will happen to your migraine if you
take estrogen replacement therapy. Usually something happens, however. The most common form of estrogen replacement therapy is the use of Premarin, which is a mixture of mul-
tiple forms of estrogen. It appears that estrogen patches, which
allow for the gradual release of estrogen, preventing precipi-
tous falls, seem least likely to worsen the problem and the most
likely to help. Other estrogen preparations may also be acceptable, particularly those which also contain male sex hormones. Look also for implantable forms, which give very even,
continuous levels, to be available in the future.

*A 28-year-old woman had migraines that were particularly se-
vere when she had her periods. She just found out that she is
pregnant. She has stopped all her medications for her headaches,
but is worried about what she can do if she gets a migraine.*

While we are on the subject of hormones, what about pregnancy? What will happen to your migraines and what can you
take to relieve them? The good news is that migraines usually,
but not invariably, improve during pregnancy, particularly in
the second and third trimesters. The bad news is we don't know
very much about the safety of drugs during pregnancy, so we
employ as many of the nonmedication methods as we can.
There are some drugs that are a particular concern for a pregnant migraine patient. Ergots can make the uterus contract,
leading to miscarriages. Divalproex sodium (Depakote) can
cause severe malformations. The simple painkillers with bu-

talbital and acetaminophen (Fioricet, Esgic) might be safe, but it is important to understand the limitations of our knowledge of drug safety during pregnancy. When we quote side effects to you, it is from well designed, scientific studies where these are measured. In pregnancy, we certainly don't test the situation purposely by giving drugs to pregnant women. Our only knowledge comes from retrospective or prospective observations of women who took them. Scientifically, this way of studying risk is flawed. Therefore, we will never be able to fully assess the safety of any drug in pregnancy.

Medication for Tension-Type Headache

Tension-type headaches are very common, but, fortunately, the chronic variety is fairly rare. The episodic ones often require little treatment and respond to relaxation or the addition of a heat pack to the back of the neck. A mild, over-the-counter, painkiller is fine to take as well. If they are more severe, they often respond to one of a host of medications that contain butalbital (Fiorinal, Fioricet, Esgic, etc.). If you take these, be aware of rebound headaches, so that you never use these more often than three times each week or more than 10 tablets each week. The major side effect is sedation, so you do not drive a care or operate a dangerous machine under the influence of these drugs. Moderate to severe tension headaches usually occur as part of the spectrum of migraine and respond best to antimigraine drugs such as triptans.

When tension-type headaches become chronic (occupy more than half your time), they become a much more difficult problem. You might want to take a painkiller every day, but all of those drugs will have unsafe side effects if you do this. The main treatments for chronic tension headaches are several drugs that are used to treat depression, tricyclic antidepressants. Whether they work has nothing to do with whether you are depressed. They are not always effective, but they are the drugs most likely to work, and they are relatively safe to take for the months and years that you may need them.

These are very difficult headaches to treat; be patient if your doctor keeps trying to adjust or change your medications. Avoid taking painkillers frequently or you will never get anywhere with your treatment. Nonmedication techniques of all kinds should be employed, including physical therapy, chiropractic therapy, massage, and exercise to increase the range of motion of the neck and shoulders to reduce local triggers in these regions. Biofeedback is a self-teaching tool where we train you to reduce the amount of muscle tension in the face, head, neck, and shoulders. This may help, particularly if you are good at mental imagery. Unfortunately, in this era of managed care, it is getting more and more difficult to get these services covered under insurance plans. Stress management programs can also be employed. The use of heat packs to the neck and shoulders makes sense, too. As with other forms of chronic pain, a regular exercise program helps control the pain through natural mechanisms.

Medication for Cluster Headache

The treatment of cluster headaches is another matter altogether. These headaches are not just a variety of migraine, and what we told you about migraine doesn't necessarily apply to cluster headaches. They are severe and disabling attacks, and every attempt should be made to treat them aggressively.

When we treat cluster headaches, we need to use both prophylactic (preventive) and abortive (acutely administered) agents. We use lithium carbonate, divalproex sodium, and verapamil most often, and sometimes a combination of these. Corticosteroids, like prednisone, work well, but have many problems associated with prolonged use, so we don't use them frequently. We only treat for the duration of the cluster, although that may be unpredictable. The best predictor is how long past clusters have lasted, but that doesn't always hold up as an absolute predictor. A drug might work well for one cluster, then fail miserably on another, so don't refuse to retry a medication that failed you in the past. Often in the beginning and toward the end of a cluster, fragments of the headaches may occur that are mild and brief. However, the discomfort is in the same location as the regular attack, so if you have cluster headaches, you recognize this only too well.

Another treatment for cluster is a drug called capsaicin applied to the inside of the nose. This is made from a hot pepper extract. With repetitive use, it depletes a pain-producing chemical called substance P. This treatment may work only after a week or more of applications. It really burns, however— so if you try it, our phone number is unlisted.

These treatments for cluster headache are preventive and, at best, will relieve only a moderate percentage of attacks. Therefore, something needs to be available for acute attacks. Painkillers, even narcotics, are quite ineffective at relieving the pain of cluster. The biggest concern with narcotics is addiction, and there aren't enough narcotics in the world to get rid of the pain of a cluster headache. Also, these headaches can occur several times a day for months, so you can imagine how many of these drugs you could wind up taking. Most important, however, is that they don't even work well.

Oxygen may work well; you need to have a large tank of pure oxygen with a special mask, breathe it in at the first sign of an attack, then continue to inhale until your headache goes away. This treatment has a fairly good success rate, doesn't make you tired, and can be administered at home or at the office. It is quite safe (unless someone smokes around it). Sumatriptan (Imitrex) by injection is amazingly effective within minutes. It is fine to try oxygen first and save the sumatriptan for headaches that don't respond to oxygen, or when you are away and don't have access to oxygen. One concern is that for an unknown reason, cluster headache patients commonly smoke and therefore have an increased risk of heart disease. Your doctor has to consider the safety issues of sumatriptan even more if you take this drug for cluster. It is interesting that oxygen treats only cluster headaches and not migraine although sumatriptan treats both.

8

What Do I Have to Look Forward To?

In the midst of a siege of migraines, it is difficult to believe the situation will ever improve. No one knows what the frequency of your headaches will be in the future. We can make some predictions, however, and they contain both good and bad news.

Migraine Prevalence Over the Life Span

The prevalence of migraine over the life span has been addressed in studies. The answer is that if you are younger than your early 40s, they are likely to get worse before they get better. If you are over this age, you are on the road to recovery. If you have tension-type headaches or cluster headaches, the chance of remission is uncertain.

It has been postulated that migraine has something to do with serotonin receptors. As we age, the number of these receptors declines. If there is something wrong with these receptors, that abnormality may also decline with age. So the best thing that you can do to cure your migraine is to age.

Studies of migraine prevalence with age show the same peak prevalence for men and women, although the number of males with migraine is much smaller after childhood. In other words, in both men and women, the number of people with migraines starts low in childhood, increases over time until the early 40s, and then begins to decline. You might conclude that menopause was the deciding factor, but there must be some other factor to explain why men have the most migraines at the same age as women do. This does not mean that hormonal factors are irrelevant. Many women with migraine become painfully aware that their problems can increase if they are given estrogen replacement therapy or take birth control pills. But men don't do this, so there must be another explanation.

Avenues of Research

Migraine treatments are advancing rapidly. There are two avenues of research: better medications to stop and prevent attacks, and ways of curing migraine. We now are developing a biochemical model of migraine. With a model, experts can craft treatments to alter biochemical pathways and neurotransmitters. Without a model, predictions of what might work are primitive and nonspecific.

We never had an animal model of any kind of headache to help guide research. We assume that rats don't get migraines, but if we are wrong, they certainly can't report that they are feeling better with treatment. But models of serotonin receptors can be drawn on a computer, and molecules can be designed that may create changes to affect headache. This goes beyond depending on someone to report whether a treatment seems beneficial.

In the nineteenth century, Liveing noted that megrim occurred within families. In 1994, the first gene for a rare type of migraine, *familial hemiplegic migraine* was identified. A second gene, located near the first on the same chromosome was recently identified. Current genetic studies suggest that channels transporting certain ions in the brain may be defective in migraineurs and somehow interfere with serotonin release or impair the ability to stop a migraine once it is triggered. It does appear that migraine is associated with more than one gene, and we are not ready to begin fixing these genetic abnormalities directly to cure migraine. Recognizing that a tendency toward migraines is inherited should not make you feel hopeless. There is still much that can be done to modify the expression of headaches in the individual.

Patients often say, "How could this problem be genetic, since I just developed it last year?" Perhaps migraine genes, while always present, are expressed only at certain times in your life. Many cases of balding, Huntington's disease, and perhaps the fundamentals of aging may be programmed in our genes, but express themselves at specific time points in the life cycle.

Genetic problems often remain in a population if they confer some advantage for the survival of the species. For example, there is a high prevalence of the gene for sickle cell disease in Africa, which often leads to painful bouts of crisis. However, such gene carriers have an increased immunity to developing malaria, which might otherwise be a fatal infection. Migraineurs are very sensitive to lights, sounds, and smells. They seem to be excessively in touch with their environment. That trait has made many migraineurs very successful people in other aspects of life. Perhaps in prehistoric days, those with migraine were more likely to anticipate an attack by predators and were therefore better able to escape and survive long enough to have children who carried that gene.

Genetic researchers are interested in comorbidity that runs in families. Comorbid conditions that occur in families may indicate genetic abnormalities located close together on the chromosome. As we approach the era of gene therapy, this information becomes very important.

The more we know about the chemistry of headaches, the easier it will be to design drugs that target the abnormalities that cause the problems. These new agents should be safer and more effective.

9

Here's the Take-Home Message

We hope you have concluded that if you have headaches, it is not your fault. If you are depressed, you should understand that you aren't depressed because you have headaches, nor do you have headaches because you are depressed.

Get the care you need. It is you who are suffering and losing time out of your life. Give a treatment program time, but if it is not working, change the program. Don't hesitate to change doctors and get specialty care if you are not doing well. Make certain your doctor really understands the impact that the headaches are having on your life.

Make sure that revisits are scheduled regularly. Periodic examinations and medication adjustment are needed. Headaches don't always remain the same. There will be times of your life when they will change, and your treatment has to change. This is not always for the worse. Migraines, for example, may begin to improve on their own, and your requirements for preventive medication are expected to change. Your medical status may also change, and some of these changes may affect your headache management. If you develop high blood pressure or heart disease, medications that you may use for your migraine may no longer be safe or appropriate. Aging is often associated with the development of new medical problems. Be suspicious of care where one treatment is promoted for all headache problems. You should understand by now that there are many type of headaches.

One thing you certainly can do, not just for yourself, but for others, is to continue to learn what is going on in headache research and treatment. You can teach others what you know so that they don't have to live with misinformation. You can also teach others with this problem how to live better with it. That includes avoiding some of the pitfalls that can make it worse. When you get older and find that this plague is yours no longer, you still have a responsibility to help educate those who are suffering.

Support groups can be very helpful. They all need knowledgeable leaders and members. Who said ignorance is bliss? If you are uninformed, your medical care won't be as good as you might wish, and you may find that you don't take advantage of things that you can do to prevent and better treat your headaches.

One day, chronic headaches may become curable, not just manageable.

Then we will write a new edition of this book.

Index